Chloé Pierre is the Black female founder of thy.self, which she was inspired to launch in October 2018 after struggling to find a space that resonated with her within wellness. Chloé's mission is to make wellness more approachable and accessible to the people that it's origins are derived from. Chloé started her career working in fashion PR and over the last decade, has expanded her experience into marketing, where she serves as a Digital Marketing Consultant for some of the biggest global brands including Nike Jordan, BBC and H&M. *Take Care* is her debut book.

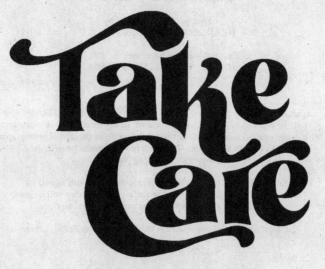

CHLOÉ PIERRE

HEADLINE

First published in 2023 by
HEADLINE PUBLISHING GROUP

First published in paperback in 2024 by
HEADLINE PUBLISHING GROUP

1

Cataloguing in Publication Data is available from the British Library

ISBN 978 1 4722 8603 1

Typeset in Monticello by CC Book Production

Printed and bound in Great Britain by Clays Ltd, Elcograf S.p.A.

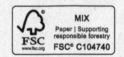

Headline's policy is to use papers that are natural, renewable
and recyclable products and made from wood grown in well-managed forests
and other controlled sources. The logging and manufacturing processes
are expected to conform to the environmental regulations
of the country of origin.

HEADLINE PUBLISHING GROUP
An Hachette UK Company
Carmelite House
50 Victoria Embankment
London EC4Y 0DZ

www.headline.co.uk
www.hachette.co.uk

To my community. This book is for YOU, women like you everywhere and our people. I couldn't have done it without you, and I definitely wouldn't do it for anyone else. May this experience guide you into knowing who you are, taking care of yourself, helping you to discover what you can achieve at any time in this life and knowing how to be at one with all that is you.

Blessings ✿

CONTENTS

CONTENTS

INTRODUCTION

My own personal wellbeing journey came about because I realised I didn't know how to take care of myself. Common phrases like 'take care' and 'be well' just seemed like polite small talk, something I often participated in myself. It's the culture, right?! I didn't actually have any idea what the fundamentals of these common phrases truly meant – what it is to be well or to take care, what that might actually look like in action, or even how to respond beyond just saying 'will do, thanks!' Thinking back to it now, if I'm keeping it real, even that answer was an absolute lie – I probably wasn't actually taking that much care of myself, and instead just wanted to keep it moving, as did the person who said it also, I'm sure. Now that I'm older though, I've found myself starting to dig deeper into even how our language hints at or evokes the concepts of wellness and how we *still* so often take it for granted.

Growing up, I was pretty much taught that to be well was to be primarily concerned with the physical – a state of being that would be recognisable to those around you based purely on your external appearance, with bonus points if you're able to talk about it out loud. But after a while, fuelled by my own feelings and by things happening in the world around me, my personal view of my exterior facade began crumbling. It became more and more noticeable to others, too. By that point, I realised that the more external shift was aligning pretty well with the nonsense that was going on internally in my mind at the time. I was lonely, unfulfilled, hurt, broken, confused, destructive, angry, unkind, damaged, susceptible to injury, viruses and medical issues. I was a total mess, and I had to own that. Not only did I not like myself, but I also didn't even really know who I was. You know when someone asks you to describe yourself and you don't know what to say or where the question begins and ends? Am I supposed to be selling myself here or answering truthfully based on how I feel? And to be honest, either way, I came up dry.

I started to spend more time alone with myself – and when I say alone, I mean actively choosing to sit in spaces of utter loneliness and silence – and during that period, I realised that unlike all the things I had been told growing up about appearances and aesthetics, wellness and well-being were inner jobs. Saying that now in 2022 doesn't feel like the most radical realisation by any means; I think it's something we're all coming to know and understand more broadly, but I still find myself asking, do we really know it? Do we embody it? Do we recognise and appreciate the true feeling of being well? Can you point it out in a line-up? Can we control it? Can we manifest it? Are we beholden to it? I don't have the answers to these questions for you, or even for myself really, but I think they'll differ for us all. Some will ring true more than others, but even thinking of the answers right now is still a challenge, I'll tell you that.

I recently watched and rewatched and then hopped on Spotify to replay *The Diary of a CEO* podcast by Steven Bartlett and his interview with Jordan Peterson called 'How To Become The Person You've Always Wanted To Be'. In it, he mentioned the sometimes unbearable job of finding self, and I'm paraphrasing, but the gist of it was that you have to be desperate for it. He talks about the suffering of being lost as something that ruins us to our core, making us harmful to ourselves and others, incapable of nurturing good, healthy relationships. This idea that as we wander around untethered, we're somehow able to find evil everywhere except in our own hearts, and that instead we should be asking ourselves: what's one thing I'm doing wrong, that I know I'm doing wrong, that I could fix, that I *would* fix? From that starting point, he says, 'Meditate on that. You will get an answer, and it won't be the one you want, but it will be the necessary one.' When I heard that, it hit me like a ton of bricks.

It hit me because I really feel like whether you're business minded or whether you're not interested in that sort of stuff at all, questions like those are where the wellness journey begins. From places of despair, desperation and self-hate, followed by looking inward with a big old microscope. And I say that because I've lived it! The pain of finding 'self' was unbearable, long-winded, isolating and uncertain, because there still aren't enough resources or spaces for people who look, sound, act and want (in that order) all the things I aspire to be, making it all somewhat uncharted territory. At the same time of course, it was also rewarding because not only did I find self, and then thy.self, but a few years further down the line, the opportunity to create this book then landed in my inbox. While I did manifest it somewhat, it wasn't at the forefront of my dreams and goals of 2020. Because whew, that year was purely about survival . . . but I overcame all of that through sheer strength. I had to do it by myself, and it was hard. But I really hope that with the publishing of this book, for you, the reader, we can spark a wave of guidance for others who want to do the same, too. Finding and facing your own truths and inadequacies is a natural but challenging part of self growth, but it is in your plan, I just know it. And that plan can start now, with the help of this book should you so decide. That decision is yours, and I'd really love for you to pause on that now.

Okay, you're back? Good! We've just covered our first lesson.

Now let me just say right now, writing this book scared the hell out of me – in so many ways and for so many reasons. The thoughts kept swimming around in my head like 'who the hell do I think I am writing this book?', 'I didn't invent wellness', 'I *never* said I was the gatekeeper of Black wellness or diversity in wellness', 'you aren't Audre Lorde, sis (sheeeeeeeet)'. I have to admit it, I do suffer from Imposter Syndrome (a lasting impact of the experience I briefly skimmed over above, and something I'll cover in depth in just a few chapters) and the force was *strongggg* with this one, especially as I started to cobble together the first few paragraphs of this book – unfortunately that's just how my mind thinks and works.

Even in this moment, while writing this book, I felt and had to contend with feeling like a fraud on more than one occasion. Writing this book and having the opportunity to do so had thoughts popping into my mind, voices mocking me, about I don't know everything there is to know about wellness or about every facet of Black women's experience – as if we're that simple to define, that we're all the same, and life itself is such an individual experience, I couldn't possibly advise everyone on every part of theirs. I had to face the truth ... I don't have all the answers, and while the pressure – the one I've placed on myself – to be able to help women like me, especially Black women like me, is real, I can't solve this alone and nor am I meant to. I'm just a young Black woman from the London region of the UK (Hackney to be exact) who had enough of feeling shit and embodying the meaning of lost. Of constantly sabotaging myself and living this disruptive life. Of feeling unwell – not in the medical sense, but holistically and mentally unwell – and living a life surely not made for anyone, let alone myself. But then, I decided to do something about it, and I'll share what I did in great detail throughout this book.

If you've just opened this book for the first time, I'm guessing ... wildly, that this too, is the point you're also at. You may feel tired, frustrated, overwhelmed, uninspired, and truly, we could go on and on, but greater than how you are feeling right now and the synonyms you can vocalise, can we just conclude that enough is enough? It's okay to say, 'I am a beautiful, bold, strong Black woman, but yes, I too am tired. I have had enough. I don't want to be strong anymore', and be heard. And do something about it.

So, what did I do next?

After a while of addressing my issues and concerns through a wellbeing approach – visiting as many women's circles, accessing wellbeing spaces as a form of therapy, going to the gym, researching wellbeing in its entirety *thanks to Web2*, discovering more aligned rituals that didn't stereotype my ancestry, experimenting with spiritual awareness and understanding – my awareness of these 'wellbeing' spaces heightened, and I very soon realised that I was often the only Black, plus-sized person in the room. At times, I felt the privilege in a positive sense and was soooo pleased I had reached this point in my life, in my career, but then came a feeling of resisting this idea of privilege, which meant only one of my kind could be able to experience this. After all, I didn't believe I was that special, especially not against my own kind, my own visions. So, from then on, my experiences in these spaces became clouded with frustration, to the point of me becoming very uncomfortable with myself in said spaces. I had to stop myself and figure out why was this happening, asking myself why these seemingly inclusive spaces were even upholding whitewashing ideals. Then I would venture to what I believed was the safety and privacy of my mobile phone and personal research only to be overwhelmed by

> 'We live in a disempowering time'
> – Sheila Atim

similar companies on the internet shoving the idea that my complex wellness and self-care dreams would all be fulfilled simply by buying their products and being served the same ads over and over again seconds after mentioning something really similar (don't get me started on the privacy side of things). Ultimately, after wading through all this information and trying to decipher these red-herring solutions, I thought to myself, what if the choices I make throughout my life on a day-to-day basis – including how to survive and to choose joy in all its forms – *are* wellness? It's not exactly rocket science, but you know what? It worked.

After taking wellness into my own hands, every day ... choosing myself and my opinions meant that I felt better about the choices I was making to live my life for me, and I continued that practice every day as if it was my religion and spiritual choice. Then I thought to myself, 'I can't be alone in this struggle to figure my life out and strive to be well. If no one cracked the code for me, maybe the least I can do is help make the process easier for someone else going through the same thing.' And so I created an Instagram account under the name thy.self, sharing the kind of content and representative imagery that I wished I had seen during my own rough patches and while growing up: the exploration of luxury wellness spaces and research into the meaning of wellness through the eyes of Black and Brown women. Then, without realising it, thy.self as we know it today was born.

Simply put, thy.self is a disruptive wellness brand, challenging the norms of what wellness looks like, diversifying the wellness industry and actualising self-care and self-love in an inclusive and relatable way. I was inspired to first create this community because I believe the wellness industry is nowhere near where it needs to be when it comes to inclusivity and approachability, so we needed a community to support the mission.

Since thy.self's conception in October 2018, it's been steadily growing into the early stages of a brand that wants to disrupt and challenge the community in which it takes up space: creating a platform to allow people the space, freedom and accessibility of health and wellness, with the help of our community. Many of whom will hopefully be reading this right now. You know who you are – I LOVE YOU! Thank you for sticking by me, supporting me, mentioning thy.self in new spaces and for keeping us/me going.

The thy.self community is made up of like-minded modern people who are conscious of the need to be able to share their vulnerabilities, strengths and coping mechanisms with other self-identifying women and people like them. thy.self unapologetically connects women and people of all ages through genuinely positive self-care initiatives, self-love discussions and positive awareness. We believe in actualising self-care, discovering what 'loving ourselves' actually means, how it is seen in our society, how it benefits our lives, tackling extremely tough subjects affecting the community and the modern world and figuring out the role that self-love and prioritising wellbeing can play in helping with this. It's about supporting and educating ourselves and others on the IRL applications of these theories that have so often felt out of reach for us.

Now I get to share this concept with you all, my

community, every single day, and that brings me more joy than you can imagine.

Audre Lorde wrote in *The Transformation of Silence into Language & Action*: 'It is important to share how I know survival is survival and not just a walk through the rain.' And now here I am, writing a book that will allow me to share my learnings *and* the learnings of icons, rising stars and Black women all around the world (some you may know already and others will be a welcomed revelation). From here on out, we will have our very own Black Wellness manifesto – a guide for Black women everywhere to assist them on their personal wellness journey. This book, this guide, is one that we can hold on to for life and one that you can ultimately curate, too. After all, wellness is a deeply personal journey, one without a destination or a certain end point.

So, why now? In truth, and within the confines of this safe space we are building together through this book, I feel comfortable saying what you probably know too. The

'When I dare to be powerful – to use my strength in the service of my vision – then it becomes less and less important whether I am afraid,'
– Audre Lorde,
The Transformation of Silence into Language & Action

world has been changing, and the battle of ugliness, truth and hope is incredibly real. For the first time in many people's lifetime, Black women's voices and stories are being heard, and these stories, our culture, our being, are more valuable than ever. We are living in a time our ancestors, even as close as our grandparents, could never have dreamt of. As a community, we are moving towards an unknown territory – one we have the power to shape – and individually, we are no longer glossing over or shamefully hiding our mental health or our challenges, and instead, we are speaking up about the inequalities, the feelings of inferiority, the struggle for equality, the abuse, the pain and the negligence that manifests itself as a result of these systems that didn't and still don't serve us – whether that's through medical racism, institutional racism, lack of representation everywhere, power dynamics in our homes and the states of our homes and families, our minds, our bodies, Imposter Syndrome, anxiety disorders, sis, go ahead . . . you name it.

And you know why that is? It would be easy to say that we've just had enough or that we as a community are collectively tired, but in truth, I think those things have been the case for a while now. Instead, I think this shift stems from something else that we may not even realise about ourselves. We have begun to see each other, not just what we look like, but we recognise ourselves in each other and our communal experiences, regardless of where on Earth we are currently situated. We can finally see each other, and we are not afraid to embrace or support each other publicly. We are joining arms in our commonalities. We are lifting each other up – even if it is just by sharing each other's accomplishments, work, experiences, names and stories on the 'gram. We aren't holding on to our current locations and bases as a way of identifying or separating ourselves from each other. The diaspora is truly alive! We are doing so much, collectively and individually, to free ourselves from both visible and invisible confines, and finally the world has cottoned on, borne witness and started to *finally* acknowledge our collective power and followed our lead. At times, we may feel as if this is an allowance, and that to take the mic means we have borrowed time to amplify our voices, but if we really stop to take in all of this change, we don't need anyone's approval. We ourselves are the majority, despite what we are told or the language we are implored to use, and we follow our own lead. No questions asked.

Do you realise what we have created? What we have started and why it means we actually can't stop now? What we have started is a movement, yes, but it's more than that. This is the legacy and the generational wealth you hear of. It isn't just for the families and communities we reside in; it's for us all. It's us saying: we exist and we exist loudly. We believe in ourselves. We believe in each other. We have a story, and most importantly, we take care of ourselves.

There is no way we could discuss a topic like this without raising the experience of 2020 – the loss and tragedy of George Floyd. Not only did it rip our hearts out, like I said above, but also, we were heard, for what felt like the first time. We felt the pain collectively and spoke out. It resounded through the world, and even if this isn't the change we want to see all at once, it's change and a step forward. We have to believe that. None of this should be taken for granted. So, if we continue with the same energy, won't we change the future for our children and those who come after them?

No longer is being educated and successful separate

> 'Life is very short. What we have to do must be done in the now.'
> – Audre Lorde, The Transformation of Silence into Language and Action

from or something that needs to be prioritised over our wellbeing. And no longer is wellness something we can keep separate from our culture and our joy. It is bundled into everything we are and everything we do, and in many ways, it forms the positive boundaries which protect us on our journey and how we move through the world. What we can dream of and what we can achieve are both intrinsically linked to our capacity and ability, which is a direct product and indication of how well we are.

So, the truth is, sometimes I still feel like an imposter, depending on what challenges I'm up against and, to be quite honest, the Lord does give me them in good measure. Trust! But I keep pushing myself, I keep moving, I keep trying and I keep doing things. And I do it knowing that in my very existence, good or bad, I'm doing so to honour my ancestors, my community and future generations, hoping to make them proud of the work I've done. It's my mission to continue to learn and discover more and more about people, our people, their work, experiences, their teachings, digest that and then share it back with our people. What I have learnt from my own experiences of wellness is that our stories are incredibly important. They help us and our community reclaim our identity and build something new – something even more magnificent than we've had before.

We get to turn those lost pieces of our heritage that may have been taken from us or erased in the past and transform them into self-care, wellness and wisdom.

As it says in the dedication, I wrote this book for our people. Yes, it's written in my Black British voice, tone, language, grammar and all the rest of it, but I want it to be for all of us. With this book, I want to reclaim our lost legacy of wellness and bring it back to the forefront and that's something I believe we can do together. By reading and holding this book to your heart like you would a rose quartz crystal, I hope that you will be reminded of your strength, reminded of your resilience and reconnected with your personal reserve of power and love of self. This book will also serve to remind you that you are not alone. You are one of many great, powerful, mystical people, and you deserve to be well.

> 'The love expressed between women is particular and powerful because we have had to love in order to live; love has been our survival.'
> – Audre Lorde, Sister Outsider: Essays and Speeches

And, despite the focus I place on Black women at the heart of what I do, I am a firm believer in #WellnessForAll, which you will see plastered across most, if not all thy.self material. I just wanted to start with my people, which is where my heart centres, first and foremost. There hasn't always been a space for this, but I unapologetically disregard that.

This book is and can be for everyone and anyone interested in wellness, whether you're in need of it personally or whether you earnestly want to see positive change for those who unfortunately were never given much hope of this. Whether you are a parent of a Black or mixed-race child or your partner or their family is Black or your friendships or other relationships include Black people or you simply wish to gift or donate this to someone you think could draw positive sentiment from the subject and practice of wellness, please feel free and welcome here. Hell, take ownership and dish out reparations in this way, I for one won't be mad at it.

Money from the book sales I receive personally will be shared among charities including Black Minds Matter UK, used for the amplification of wellness research for Black people and to support thy.self activations created specifically for the demographic highlighted in this book – Black women.

This book aims to open your eyes, navigate the disconnect and sharpen your understanding of the Black experience when it comes to wellbeing, teaching you how to care for it from whichever position you stand and hopefully help you push for change. This book is about good choices, period. Like nearly every industry you could possibly name, the wellness industry has long failed to consider the Black experience. With your own research, it won't take long to discover that many industries still do this. It's intentional, of course. But so am I, and we'll unpack this together, and in the process, empower each other.

This book is not intended to be a substitute for

professional advice, diagnosis, medical treatment or therapy. As a wellbeing advocate, I will always advise my audience to seek the advice of qualified medical and mental health providers, and go to them with any questions you may have (exceptionally big or exceptionally small) regarding any mental health symptoms or medical conditions new and old.

I'd like you to treat this book less like a book and more like an encyclopedia of our wellness and heritage combined or, even better, a friend, a family member or the companion of truth you've been looking for your whole life. If this manifesto of thoughts and insight into Black female wellness found its way into your life, know that it is for a reason and that it's meant to be. We are an extremely well-connected tribe regardless of location, country of birth, language we speak, complexion of skin, shape of our hips, kink of hair or where we are in our journey.

Finally, what I want to share with you is one practice, which even I overlook sometimes, but I often say to myself and now to you ... whoever you are, wherever you are: *'Your wellbeing does matter, sis. Take care of yourself first!'*

One

WHAT IS WELLNESS?

'To me, wellness means checking in on myself and the different stages of my mental and physical health. If I'm not asking myself questions, it means I'm not good, I'm not doing well. Wellness for me is about the approach to taking care of oneself.'

– Enam Asiama

The question 'what is wellness?' is the one that set me on my personal journey to discover the real meaning of wellness. Such a simple word, it was still so hard to pin down and understand, even when typed into Google. The Global Wellness Institute defines wellness as the 'active pursuit of activities, choices and lifestyles that lead to a state of holistic health'. The institute believes that wellness is often confused with terms such as health, wellbeing and happiness. While there are common elements among them, wellness is not distinguished by referring to a static state of being (e.g. being happy, in good health or a state of wellbeing). Rather, wellness is associated with an active process of being aware and making choices that lead toward an outcome of optimal holistic health and wellbeing.

This definition just didn't have the impact or depth that I was desperately searching for, nor did other definitions encompass the strong feelings and understanding I have for wellness today. I felt it didn't hold the answers to the things I was facing, or even give me the tools to help me find those answers for myself. What's worse is that within this confusing, contradictory space, all that I *could* see were these arm-long lists of articles that spoke about wellness in language like 'Here are the 7 Dimensions of Wellness' or 'Five-Step Guide To . . .', but as soon as you click through, you realise each one of these 'easy steps' is complex enough to be a lifelong journey. Whether you're thinking about just your physical wellness and the energy and dedication it takes to monitor and nurture that, or occupational wellness and the years we spend pushing forward to figure out our careers, or emotional wellness, which can feel totally stable one day and miles away the next, I soon realised that wellness in many ways is everything we do. It touches every section of our lives and is a continuous practice, not a goal to be achieved.

The next hurdle of my wellness investigation was the imagery. Not to say that I ever had a specific picture in mind when I thought about wellness to begin with, but if I had, it would have been nothing like what was fed to me by my searches. These rows and rows of pristine, corporate, over-styled, boring, grey images and wordy #LiveLaugh-Love infographics with swirly text and flowery clip art. Piles of beauty products positioned as problem-solvers and a very clear and obvious demographic of who wellness is meant to be for. And guess who those people were? To be completely honest with you, as I scrolled and scrolled, I could not find a single image of a Black woman, man or child. And that didn't sit well with me, at all.

When I think of what it is to be 'well', I naturally imagine colour, vibrancy, joy, images relating to an overall visual sense of thriving. To me, wellbeing is about the things that can inspire us, uplift us and really make us believe that it's possible to turn our lives around. I see wellness as a way of life that brings us closer to our best selves and allows us to live in that technicolour. So, I really struggled to wrap my head around this depiction of it as muted, toned down and, frankly, pale as hell.

Even when you think of the origins of what we now consider mainstream Western wellness practices and ingredients – herbalism, yoga, apothecary, meditation, smudging and Cacao ritual meditation, to name a few – these rituals are derived from such rich and diverse corners of the Earth that you'd expect the imagery to reflect that too. For example, take herbalism or plant medicine, a well-known and important part of African traditional medicine and culture. Gotu Kola, a native plant in Africa that can be taken in capsule, tincture, powdered or tea form, is said to assist with stress support and depression, much like a number of plants historically found in the motherland.

People of different complexions, from different backgrounds, different shapes, different bodies and abilities have formed and created practices that fall under the umbrella of wellness. So, surely health and wellness are not exclusive to slim, white, cis men and women?

Nowadays, thanks to the internet and a society more globalised and accustomed to topics such as mental health and wellness, you can stumble upon conversations about wellness across a whole host of platforms, led by a variety of different people. You'll find pockets of TikTok dedicated to health, routines, meditation and exercises that can aid you on that journey. Instagram is filled to the brim with infographics on steps you can take and entire profiles dedicated to passing that knowledge on. Twitter threads and articles are shared that dig deep into the origins of wellness and ask some of the same questions that I'll be posing here in this book. In the public-run media, there's no shortage of possibilities to describe what wellness might be, what it might look like from person to person or how it might feel once you find it. However, the sheer volume of information now can feel both overwhelming and confusing. Because of this, I want to go right back to the source (or first recorded one) so we can streamline the information and get a clearer grasp on it.

It shocked me to discover that the term was first recorded in and recognised by the *Oxford English Dictionary* in 1654. This was during the time of William Shakespeare and Oliver Cromwell and not long before the Great Plague. Not exactly what you might think of when you imagine wellness. However, anthropological studies of ancient history reveal that the act of taking care of oneself and practices of self-actualisation and fulfillment have been around as long as humans have been on this Earth. In fact, wellness can be found in every religion that focuses on harmony of the spirits and the body and can be traced back as far as

3000 BC. You can see the foundations for modern wellness being laid in ancient Chinese, Roman and Greek history, just without the label of what we know it to be today.

The fact that the word 'wellness' was created and defined by self-professed intellectuals in the Western world in the 1600s, and then firmly embedded in its modern sense by Halbert L. Dunn in 1961 (known as one of the 'fathers of the wellness movement', hmm), displays how much a long, diverse and rich history has been co-opted through a Western, and ultimately European, lens. When it comes to wellness, we have to look outside of and beyond the definitions provided to us by dominant powers from history. The endlessly vast history of practices that have been passed down through generations is so rich, diverse and powerful and encompasses us so much more than those who have capitalised on it and flipped it for profit in recent times. Wellness is inherent in all of us, and it's our right to seek it out and form our own thoughts and opinions on it. To be well is not a privilege reserved for the rich or the white, European or even the English-speaking; it's how we all can and should (be able to) live.

In the same way it has impacted humanity for centuries, race relations has impacted the perceptions of wellness. Now, you may think it's perhaps too soon to be jumping straight into the race relations segment of this discussion, but with that being the driving force of my studies, my work, my ambitions and, yes, this book, it is and will always be a huge part of the gaze that I view the world with. The dominant identities (being white, European, male, cisgendered, heterosexual and able-bodied) have long had control over what is considered the norm. The world has been organised in a way that benefits these dominant identities and impacts how everyone with alternative identities moves through life every day. We have to acknowledge these systems and ideologies when it comes to wellness, because the disparity between the dominant identities that hold the power and those of us who hold less power or are powerless, exists here, too. It's important we don't back down when acknowledging how these structures and institutions can seek to deny Black people, Black women and people of colour as a whole of their credit, humanity and, ultimately, their peace, as a result of lack of access, appropriation, exclusion or just plain straight-up erasure. Resistance is taking back what was stolen and embracing it in both its current and former glory.

Wellness as we know it now has been boiled down into this neat little description that focuses on 'the state of being in good health, especially as an actively pursued goal', and for many people, that's totally true. But I'd love for us all to explore and come to an understanding that wellness as an umbrella term in and of itself is very complex and can differ for each and every person on this planet, just as its and our combined histories suggests. It's not going to look the same across class, location, job, gender, upbringing, sexuality or any unique combination of those intersections.

I also want to acknowledge that wellness is so much more than words or products. There's no moisturiser you can use or supplement you can take that will solve all your problems. Nor is there one magical inspirational quote, article or, shit, even book that you can read that will reprogramme you to operate at your optimal capacity.

That's why this book doesn't aim to tell you what wellness is but instead it aims to guide you with a nurturing hand on your journey through it and all of its different facets. To show you what it can mean for you, that it can mean something different to you than it does to others, regardless of how close or seemingly similar you might think you are, and that's okay. In fact, it's great and proves that the world is made of individuals, not followers, not copies of human beings, and that in itself is the beauty of the human race. I think that wellness is a hand that is not often readily available, offered or stretched out for Black women in a way that sees us fully, appreciates us or wants the best for us. Often, we're not considered in this and many other bubbles, and even when we are, we're an afterthought or misunderstood, misrepresented or made to feel that there is only room for one of our 'kind'. This book is one thing among many others that hopes to change that.

This is a guide to enable you to voice your own version of what wellness means to you and create an understanding of wellness that will serve you and the community you call your own, hopefully for a long time to come. That's the kind of generational wealth that I seek for myself, my loved ones, my family, my community, Black women everywhere and specifically for you reading this right now. This is where change starts.

I make a point of saying this at every talk we do for thy.self, on every podcast appearance and in every conversation, regardless of who it's with – when it comes to wellness, activism and change: movements are never built by one person. For me to see the changes that I want to see in my own daily life for myself and for other people who look like me, we need all hands on deck. Or at least some more. That's why this isn't about competition; it's about strength in numbers.

For some of us, wellness is not something we've bothered to think about or, should I say, been afforded the opportunity to do so. That's something I heard a lot when I was first launching thy.self, a result of the pressures placed on us to support others, to raise households, to put ourselves last out of love for those around us or even stemming from these small, diminishing voices in our own head that tell us we're overreacting or being dramatic when it comes to the discussion of our health, both physical and mental. For some, it's a feeling they chase, a goal they try to work towards in bursts when they can or a process of growth and transformation in the face of change.

When I think of wellness, however, I see it as an inner strength that we are all born with access to, an awareness – a birthright, dare I say – a continuous lifestyle without any particular end goal in mind. I think in Western societies and under capitalism, we are always taught that there needs to be an end goal to everything we do. It's the mindset that if you are the right person, who does the right things, buys the right tools, goes to the right classes and most importantly just tries hard enough, then you'll get there. Capitalist companies are reinforcing this message. They tell us and sometimes manipulate us to believe wellness is something you can buy. This multi-billion-pound industry supplies us with an endless number of ways to empty our pockets in search of the ultimate feeling of being well.

Ultimately, wellness does not need to cost money, and it definitely does not need to be expensive. In fact, some of the most influential practices within it literally stem from communities that preach and live the exact opposite principles to capitalism.

Now that we've interrogated wellness, I believe that, in summary, wellness is way too personal to be definitively nailed down in one sentence or even by one person. It's an individual process that can be shared with others in moments but ultimately encapsulates the physical, emotional, spiritual, behavioural, religious, nutritional and many other aspects of your life. It's a lifestyle that is constant and ever-changing, a lot like the world around us and all the other people in it too.

I truly believe that with patience, wellness is a journey of great beauty and deep meaning that can be travelled by us all. It's something that many of us crave but only a few are able to open themselves to and even fewer have the tools to access. It's something we can call our own, and for Black women in particular, it's something we can reclaim simply by observing it, practising it and owning the facets of it that are already embedded in who we are, our DNA, our melanin, our very existence today. Wellness can be a tool to build ourselves higher than the treatment we receive and the circumstances we find ourselves in.

'Until the lion learns how to write, every story will glorify the hunter.'
– African proverb

So, why do we need to define and document wellness,

specifically through the lens of Black women's experience? Or, in other words, why does a book like this need to exist? Despite having to navigate the 'strong Black woman' trope and perceptions on a daily basis, figures and data simply don't lie. In 2021, the BBC reported that in the UK alone, government figures year on year report that Black women are more likely than white women to experience common mental health problems, such as anxiety and depression. As this book is in the process of being written, there is finally a research project underway, diving deeper into depression in Black women, but this is likely to be the first time you hear of such a study. Shout out to Anna of BIWD Study.

And what about the global Black female community? Should we not consider them too? As well as this, sectioning powers under the Mental Health Act also end up disproportionately affecting Black people too.

For those unaware of what 'sectioning' actually means: it's when you are kept in a hospital under the Mental Health Act 1983 due to mental health concerns that are deemed severe or a potential danger to yourself or others. There are different types of sections, each with different rules to keep you in hospital. The length of time, treatment and care that occurs during your time in hospital also depends on which section you are detained under, as well as your personal circumstances.

When it comes to Black women, we literally face risks to our health as a result of the discrimination that we face

---

* Gov.uk, 'Common mental disorders', 2017

out in the world – both from health professionals who don't take our concerns seriously and from the biological and psychological wear and tear caused by the chronic stress of what is sometimes just merely existing.

> 'The most insidious kind of prejudice is found where many least expect it – at the heart of respectable society.'
> – Reni Eddo Lodge

What we need to understand and eventually action ourselves as Black women – because Lord knows who else will do it for us – is that wellness, our wellness, has been historically compromised, and when you pair that with a potential lack of support, trauma of all kinds (large and small), unhealthy coping mechanisms, chronic illness, stress, disability, substance abuse – the list goes on – the results can be pretty damning. The sooner we grasp the urgency of needing to care for our wellness above all, the sooner we can get the help we need, raise our voices, make change and begin to see a positive difference in ourselves and those around us. For far too long, we have been silenced, and collectively, we will need to admit that at times we've even silenced each other too.

As Black women, we have long been raised, programmed and expected to care for others, so the most basic notion of taking time for yourself can be seen as selfish or indulgent. But in that very basic sense, we have a revelation in front of us. That is, that self-care absolutely can be and is a Black feminist act and a necessary path that we need to uphold in order to protect our community and our futures.

TYPES OF WELLNESS

'Experts' will tell you that there are somewhere between five and eight dimensions of wellness to focus on for optimal health results, but we are living in *this* dimension and, well ... My belief is that wellness is everywhere and in everything. So, let's focus on what is real, what isn't, what serves us and what doesn't as Black women, and let's not put a number on it. Instead, I'd love to explore a few aspects of wellness that society and professionals have established and view them through the lens of Black women's experiences.

Physical Wellness

Physical wellness as a definition means caring for your body and building or maintaining physical health now and into the future. As far as we know, myself and the 'experts' can agree, a healthy body is one that is obtained through exercise, nutrition, nurture and self-care and sleep.

However, we must remember that when it comes to physical health, whole health – or as Grace Victory called it, '"whole"-istic health' – it should not be limited to a very specific vision of a person with a very specific set of boundaries. To be physically healthy is about so much more than just what size clothes you wear or how many abs are showing when you tense your muscles. Wellness is a holistic integration of physical, mental and spiritual wellbeing, fuelling the body, engaging the mind and nurturing the spirit. Although it always includes striving for health in the physical sense, it's more about living life fully and allowing yourself to become the best kind of person that your potential, circumstances, genetics and fate will allow – which we'll come to find out, as the magical beings that we are as Black women, is a potential far greater than we might initially realise.

Emotional Wellness

Emotional wellness can be understood through years of self-awareness and appreciation of the thoughts and feelings that you yourself experience, as well as those held by others around you. Understanding and respecting your feelings, values and attitudes, and also appreciating the feelings of others, learning to manage your emotions in a constructive and productive way and making a conscious choice to feel 'positive' and enthusiastic about your life and the way you live it. It might look like emotional stability in the face of chaotic circumstances, an inner peace or contentment or a strong ability to communicate through difficult situations.

Vocational Wellness

A dimension not often discussed in the wider wellness bubble, but one that accounts for much of the modern Black woman's health and ability to access healthcare, her ambitions and the trajectory of her and those close to her. All of these things are often determined by the specifics of her vocation(s) and the degrees of wellness that surround her work environment.

We spend so much of our lives working, thinking about working, avoiding working, trying to work more or less, that of course it plays an integral role in how well we are. In order to build a healthier connection to wellness in our vocations, we need to prepare for and participate in work that provides personal satisfaction and life enrichment and that is consistent with our values, goals and lifestyle, or we need at least to find ways to build that into the work–life balance that we achieve long-term. To obtain this, as Black women we must consciously seek work that contributes to our individual and unique gifts, skills and work that is personally meaningful, rewarding and, most importantly, respectful. We may have been taught that this was not possible or not on the cards that we have been dealt, but speaking from experience, not only do I believe that you can, I assure you that you can.

Spiritual Wellness

Our search for meaning and purpose in human existence is often directly correlated to religion, but don't think it has to be. Many define spirituality according to religious values, while others find expression of spirituality through personal relationships or through nature. Much like religious wellness, spiritual wellness provides us with systems of faith, beliefs, values, ethics, principles and morals, but they aren't intrinsically linked to a higher being or organised community. A healthy *spiritual* practice may simply include meditation, travel, forgiveness and expressions of compassion. Spiritual wellness can allow Black women to live a life consistent with our own beliefs outside of the cultural systems and institutions that we have historically been brought up in, nurturing something more bespoke and specific to us.

Environmental Wellness

Environmental wellness refers to your sense of safety, comfort and connection with your physical surroundings. It can be enhanced by living more in harmony with the planet and our nearest and dearest communities, because wellness in this domain begins in your immediate surroundings. Your personal space has a direct impact on your state of mind, emotional wellbeing and productivity; it's a lesson a lot of us had to learn the hard way during the years of the pandemic. This aspect of wellness explores the optimal ways to curate and maintain your personal space, how you might like to navigate through it and what you may choose to protect it from or invite into it. If we take it one step further, environmental wellness also extends beyond your personal space to larger communities, geographic areas and the rest of this floating rock too. Understanding how your social, natural and built environments affect your health and wellbeing as well as having an awareness of the unstable state of the Earth and the effects of your daily habits on the physical environment are key. How can we give back to our home (aka Earth) and foster a meaningful connection to it?

'Climate change is not just a white people problem,' Heizal Nagginda explains in the conversations she has within her Ugandan community. As people of the Earth, originally and spiritually, we must own our place in the ecosystem, voice our opinions and fight for the world we care for, on both large platforms and more intimate spaces too – for our sake and for the sake of those that will come after us. Demonstrating a commitment to a healthier planet is an overlooked dimension for Black women but one we can start now.

Financial Wellness

In the grand scheme of things, as women, it's a fairly new reality to be able to manage our finances outside of any male influence. For Black women, some may argue that, generally speaking, we have been doing this for years, just without credit and with a lot of hard work. Managing one's resources to be able to live within your means, making informed financial decisions and investments, setting realistic goals and preparing for short-term and long-term needs or emergencies is not anything new. The Black mother and matriarch has been doing this for years, alongside her many other roles, but, of course, the framework and structure has not always been the standard within our community and the ambition to do these things completely independently is also ever-growing.

Modern Black women are not only discovering financial wellness now, but we are also being invited to join in on the conversation and even confidently invest, too. It's something I hope in a decade's time is more normalised than ever before.

Financial wellness also includes being aware that everyone's financial values, needs and circumstances are entirely unique to them and being able to navigate these conversations within our own communities with or without the end goal being generational or community wealth.

Intellectual Wellness

Intellectual wellness simply means growing intellectually, maintaining curiosity about all there is to learn, valuing lifelong learning and responding positively to intellectual challenges. A well person expands her knowledge and skills while discovering the potential for sharing her gifts with others. Travelling a wellness path, you'll explore issues related to problem solving, creativity and learning and find ways to continue to challenge your brain and provoke new thoughts and ideas.

Take Care

Black Wellness

I think this could otherwise be described as Identity
Wellness or something similar. Here I intend it to mean
a strong and healthy connection to our identity and our
ethnic background. Learning about and having opportunities to immerse yourself in your heritage are famously
grounding exercises. The feeling of arriving in a country
you may have never been to but feeling like it is a return
or homecoming is a sense that resists logical explanation.
The sense of community and belonging is something that
we search endlessly for in life, and that bond that we feel
with kinfolk is a large piece of that puzzle for many.

34

Two

A HISTORY OF SELF-CARE

Tracing the origins of self-care is about as hard as trying to figure out who invented hummus. I once saw a documentary in which men from Greece, Israel and Morocco *all* claimed that hummus had originated in their home countries, and even to this day, if you Google the question, it's kind of hard to get a straight and definitive answer.

When it comes to the truest timeline on self-care within Black communities, to be perfectly honest, despite all my digging, I haven't landed on a rock-solid answer myself. To trace the history of it for someone in the diaspora probably starts by tracing their family lineage. And when I think about those of us who come from the Caribbean or our cousins over in the Americas, past a certain point, that process presents all kinds of challenges for reasons we all know. Even across the African continent, colonialism and the shift towards Western supremacy have meant that the documentation of our historic practices is often full of holes, if it's there at all, and the rest of it is slipping through our fingertips as our elders age and move on.

If we were to lean in slightly to the more readily available European translations and literature for the understanding and roots of self-care, the first things you'll find are self-care lessons entrenched in individualism, privilege, elitism, cronyism, highlighting European beauty standards, hygiene, rigid gender norms and the colonisation of traditions that we now commercially refer to as 'hot new trends' or 'discoveries'. Again, it's only a recent development that internet uproar forces the hand of these industries to give credit where credit is due and acknowledge the origins of the West's many adopted practices – from rhassoul clay to burning sage to yoga to mud baths. And often, when these routines are lifted, diluted and redistributed, they aren't even done with great accuracy or regard for sustainability. For example, experts suggesting that a lot of European yoga taught and marketed predominantly to adult women now via expensive memberships and classes is often derived from practices originally developed in India that were meant for adolescent boys, rather than moves suitable for all and anyone. We're literally being pushed to do things that aren't natural for our own bodies because of a lack of cultural context and understanding.

Like much of global history, ours has often been co-opted and repackaged purposefully to suit everyone but us (for clarity, I'm referring to Black and Brown people here). But, our existence and inclusion in the ideation of self-care, from its long history of being a radical act to transcending beyond its current image of modern luxury and capitalist drive, is abundant. I've said it many times, but unlike free delivery on certain online retailers or the card machine at your local off-licence, self-care doesn't have to have a required minimum spend.

A History Of Self-care

If you feel like you've been hearing the term 'self-care' thrown around more and more loosely over the last few years, you're absolutely right. According to Google Trends, the number of searches for 'self-care' has more than doubled since 2015, and the hashtag can conjure up anything from hotel towel headwraps and a fresh set of acrylic nails to idyllic bathroom selfies, cucumbers over the eyes . . . But self-care is all of those things and none of them at the same time.

What if I told you that there would be no term 'self-care' in the first place without the concept of post-traumatic stress disorder existing first? The term actually has medical and psychological roots, after being coined in the 1950s to describe activities that enabled institutionalised mental health patients to preserve some physical independence and self-dignity for the good of their health, i.e. undertaking simple tasks that helped nurture a sense of self-worth, such as exercising and personal grooming.

Again, this research centres Western society's chronology of self-care, but the practices that many know and love under the label today do stem from much further afield. So, why is it that so many of our traditions, exercises and cultural nuances are harvested and appropriated for their commercial elements and benefits by others before we even get the chance? You only need to remember the direct ignorance of the *New York Post* article about Sasha Obama that ran in 2016 to see just how entrenched this habit is. This article reported that Sasha had apparently copied the Kim Kardashian 'boxer braids' trend, completely erasing centuries of ancient and ancestral hair-braiding practices dating back to as early as 3500 BC.

We can trace self-care to the roots of the American Black Panther Party in the 1970s. The revolutionary organisation began promoting it as an essential part of their philosophy for the liberation of Black people, and in particular, their members and wider network. They saw it as a means of staying resilient while experiencing the repeated injuries and devastations of systemic, interpersonal and medical racism (to name just a few). By distributing food to those in need, including through a free breakfast programme for kids, creating health clinics, building structures to educate and make information accessible, the Black Panther Party put care into action in real tangible and inclusive ways for their communities. They imparted the belief and the infrastructure that placed huge importance on being well as a crucial tool for change, shifting the narrative seismically about the value of caring for oneself.

At the same time, the feminist movement was catching on to the term. To this day, a lot of the power of the contemporary wellness movement comes from a history of marginalised people reclaiming autonomy and joy over their bodies and selves that have for so long been doubted, discredited, neglected, dismissed and ultimately disrespected. Women have historically fallen squarely under that umbrella too, and the movement of reclaiming their own bodily health and strength in the 1970s was propelling them alongside their fight to be seen as equal in the eyes of the government, allowing them to be able to govern themselves. It goes without saying that women are now perhaps the most integral consumers and proponents of wellness in its best and worst forms.

Later on, self-care became a popular concept among health professionals studying workers in high-risk and emotionally taxing positions, attempting to understand how they could deal with those intense levels of stress. The belief driving this work was that one person cannot adequately take on the problems of others without taking care of oneself, a sentiment you still hear and feel from activists today: 'you cannot pour from an empty cup' might ring a bell.

And then, there's Audre Lorde. My personal *governess* of self-care. If it wasn't for Lorde's life, writings, sayings and teachings, I don't know if I would still be pushing for equality within wellness today. She is my biggest inspiration. It is truly because of her work that we can now see the necessity of self-care, alongside our grasping of it as a political and radical act in the world we live in.

Audre Lorde once described herself as a 'Black lesbian feminist warrior mother' who used her words to address sexism, classism, homophobia and racism in America. She is best known for intellectual mastery and emotional expression, as well as her poems that express anger and outrage at civil and social injustices she observed throughout her life. Even after her death, she and her vital words have continued to bloom into a guiding voice of reason for so many Black women. In particular those

> 'Caring for myself is not self-indulgence. It is self-preservation, and that is an act of political warfare.'
> – Audre Lorde, 'A Burst of Light' and Other Essays

who are on this discovery journey into self-care and community activism. Lorde's work urges Black feminists to embrace politics rather than fear it, especially in regard to the self.

'I urge each one of us here to reach down into that deep place of knowledge inside herself and touch that terror and loathing of any difference that lives there. See whose face it wears. Then the personal as the political can begin to illuminate all our choices,' Lorde says. 'Black women sharing close ties with each other, politically or emotionally, are not the enemies of Black men. Too frequently, however, some Black men attempt to rule by fear of Black women who are more ally than enemy.'

Now I want to ask you, do Black women's and Black men's self-care have to be different? What're the implications of the above quote?

It is my hope that the global Black community can come together with shared and combined goals for the future and a sustained vision of what self-care can and should look like to make life better for us all. No more and no longer should the Black woman work herself into the ground, no more shall we as a community and within our growing families perpetuate the age old saying 'we can sleep when we are dead' and no more shall we 'work twice as hard' to satisfy a capitalist society that consistently tries to keep us down. No more to any of that. Being seen as the pillars of our communities, not only do we uphold the legacy of building everyone around us up, but we also have to do the same with ourselves. And to honour and prioritise that is not indulgence – it's leadership.

To shirk the responsibilities layered on top of us and putting self-care first is to be actively anti-capitalist. It breaks boundaries, tears down stereotypes and leaves the door open for a new way of life. There's room for both activism and self-care, because in order for us all to prosper, there has to be both. This radical act should be acknowledged and actioned for the greater good of self *and* community.

THE ISSUE WITH SELF-CARE

As with anything and everything that blows up on a wide scale, there are pros and cons to self-care too. Especially when something has been altered in perception so much that it now can be seen to equal monetary success and popularity. Wellness in the realest sense, beyond the surface level, is one of those things that is deeply complex and nuanced. Let's dig into it.

What are the issues currently debated around self-care? Is it harmful? Is society's obsession with it problematic? Can it be practised incorrectly or too much?

My viewpoint is this: If you buy into a commercialised definition of anything, for example, self-care that promotes incessant pampering or relies solely on the consumption of products to achieve inner superpowers, then of course there are dangers. Commercialisation of self-care makes it exclusive and exclusivity means that it isn't accessible to everyone. That is problematic. Capitalism has transformed self-care in many ways to be an off-shoot of the self-improvement trend that wants the individual to relentlessly make themselves better – at their own expense. This idea that we always need more – need to consume more, be more, achieve more – is a key part of what makes the wheels in our society turn and is exactly what big businesses want. Self-care becomes just another way for individuals to buy things to improve their life. This means that other forms of self-care that are accessible, *free* and helpful are overlooked and replaced by other forms of wellness that are slyly narcissistic or just plain bank breaking.

Caring for yourself will not and should not look like giving in to every whim and fancy you have in the very moment you have it. When you think of caring well for a child, it's not just feeding them biscuits every time they ask and allowing them to not eat their broccoli. Just like that, self-care is about balance and sense and doing the deeper work as well as the fun stuff.

Done right, self-care is filling your own cup and having enough to share all round. Done wrong, self-care is over-filling your own cup, hoarding resources and leaving others thirsty. Or even worse than that, it's filling your cup with a liquid that lacks the ability to even hydrate you, instead it might make you feel worse. Wellness is not an aesthetic or a look. It's hard work at times. It can sometimes look like having a really difficult therapy session, where you leave feeling vulnerable, exhausted and confused. That therapy session might be hard, but it opens the way to a healthier you and might lead to the next sessions being much more honest, open and fulfilling.

We need to shed the expectations and consider the deeper meanings of wellness and self-care. If we can't do that then, yes, it can be harmful, damaging and problematic. Understanding this side of the coin is essential because being aware can enable us to avoid it or recognise when it's happening so we can change it.

SELF-CARE TODAY

Self-care is now a trillion-dollar industry encompassing everything from spa days and scented candles to reiki, yoga and gong baths. But the modern, commercial world of wellness is only one part of the self-care story, and we have to continue questioning 'who is allowed and entitled to practise it, benefit from it and how?' We aren't just a part of self-care and its story and history . . . we are it. We embody this, and we must claim and stand firm in this belief. We have to push to occupy spaces in rooms where we aren't always invited eagerly and feel no shame or guilt about doing so. We have to share our knowledge freely and accessibly with others and open the floodgates instead of gatekeeping. Where we see a need and desire, find ways to fill it ourselves, for ourselves. All of these things will take time and practice.

So often when others see you love yourself hard, their initial response is a feeling of insecurity or threat, because love draws its opposite into such stark contrast. This happens especially when you're not 'supposed' to love yourself according to society's historic standards. Instead of asking themselves 'how can I be like that?', human jealousy will sadly often spark onlookers to ask, 'how dare she?' But I really do believe that in leading by example, we can dispel preconceptions and inspire others to join the journey of wellbeing and self-care. Rediscovering the art of loving yourself and building your wellbeing is definitely a long old road, but it's one worth the uphill effort and one with infinite rewards.

SUSTAINABLE SELF-CARE

I have been spitting the lyrics of sustainable wellness among the thy.self community and to anyone who will listen for about four years now. This is probably one of the most buzzworthy terminologies ever, and I'm so here for it. Whenever something new is created in pop culture, it can take so long for the fire to light but when it eventually does, it really does spread like wildfire. The whole reason I started thy.self was to combat the toxic capitalism of self-care and wellness. It shouldn't have a negative impact on the planet. No more should the entry-points to wellness be taxable and worrisome, but instead they should be readily available to all through the knowledge that already lives out there in the world. Often for free.

As Black women, we are so used to being under-mined, patronised and underestimated when it comes to our spending power. But with that said, by their very design, marketers and retailers often prey on our insecurities and our wants. And that's where sustainable self-care comes in.

It is knowing that you are enough already, not just because you are talented and intelligent and beautiful and loved and valued, but purely because you exist. It's a practice that can involve self-awareness and gratitude, for example, but it's oh so much more than that too. Sustainable self-care is a rhythm. It involves trial and error as well as a dollop of gentleness. It's honouring the soft Black girl that exists within you while saying no to The Man and living within your means. It's being creative without reaching for your purse. It's looking at the planet you know in your bones you are entitled to live on fruitfully, while taking care of it consciously as if it was your own child. Seeing its natural value and power beyond labels and campaigns and markups. Environmental wellness and sustainable wellness truly go hand in hand.

And so, it's time to dust off the sustainability enthusiast within you and focus on living and practising self-care in a way that has longevity without stretching too far or harming our home. A way to do this could be to go on a beach clean. Enjoying the beauty of nature while doing fulfilling, meditative and committed work to improve it for others to enjoy.

Three

BLACK WOMEN AT THE FOREFRONT

For a subject as meaty and layered as this, it'd only be right to start by acknowledging some of the women who inspired me before we get into the deep stuff. This list is by no means exhaustive, but instead is just a small selection of Black women that I consider to be icons. They are smashing barriers and charging forward for all of us, both in the wellness space and across wider culture. They are redefining and leaving open to inspiration real seeds of change, and ultimately what it means to be a Black woman.

Elizabeth Uviebinené & Yomi Adegoke

This dynamic duo are a sparkling example of Black women thriving. Co-authors of *Slay In Your Lane: The Black Girl Bible*, they came out the gates centring Black women, our triumphs and our struggles and have kept that at the heart of their projects ever since. Friends-turned-business partners, they have also navigated their respective industries (finance and journalism) with unmistakable authenticity and drive, forging new paths and setting standards for those who follow.

Serena Williams

This titan really needs no introduction. But that's kind of the point of this section so I'll do one anyway. Serena Williams is a history maker, a gamechanger, a fighter and one of our greats. Not just for Black women but for *athletes* worldwide and people generally. A champion on the court, she has held the number one ranking for the longest consecutive run of weeks in history (186) and has spent the third longest amount of time at number one in the history of the Women's Tennis Association. With the pro recently announcing her retirement from the game, I couldn't help but iconise this as a public championing of #BlackGirlSoftLife after reading this comment: 'I have to focus on being a mom, my spiritual goals and finally discovering a different, but just as exciting, Serena.'

She and her sister Venus are the only tennis players in history to have been awarded four Olympic gold medals. When she reclaimed the number one spot in 2017 at the age of 35, she was the oldest woman to ever do so, and just four months after that, she gave birth to her first child. Her list of achievements is genuinely endless. Whew. Serena Williams.

Diane Abbott

I'm so glad I get an opportunity to give Ms Diane Abbott her flowers in this book. As the first Black woman ever

elected to UK Parliament and the longest-standing Black
MP in the House of Commons, her respect is absolutely
due. In a system that is notoriously (and maybe even
proudly) elitist and exclusionary, Aunty Diane has persisted
against some pretty tough conditions and has continuously stood her ground on issues that matter to her. Even
through the rougher patches of her path, she's shown such
strength and pushed through to the other side, winning
her constituencies with landslide votes. And to close, lest
we forget Ms Diane indulging in an M&S mojito tinnie on
the Overground line. We stan a wellness queen.

June Sarpong

Beyond just being such a ray of sunshine, June Sarpong
showed so many of us that we had a voice and a place within
the world through her visibility in broadcasting. Working
her way from a start in radio to daytime TV, she's been a
steady, joyous presence throughout our lives and holds such
a special place in Black British history, especially for us
women who follow in her footsteps in some way. To this day,
she still plays a huge part in ensuring the next generation
of broadcasters and journalists are equipped with the tools
they need to succeed, and that true representation remains
at the core of the BBC's mission too through her work as
Director of Creative Diversity.

Take Care

Nicole Crentsil

If you don't know about Black Girl Fest (BGF), I don't know for you, I really don't. As one of the co-creators of the festival, Nicole Crentsil is an absolute force, a movement and a gamechanger.

Inspiring and uplifting a new generation of Black girls through mentorship, access, resources, community and, let's be honest, pure enjoyment, BGF is an entity that really does what it says on the tin. For Black women, by Black women. Outside of that work, Crentsil is also a huge advocate and advisor for angel investment in new, refreshing businesses and has played a role in helping launch some really incredible companies and concepts too, like Ruka hair for example. If someone is in the know and using those superpowers for good, it's Nicole.

Sharmadean Reid

One of the most visible Black women in the entire UK beauty industry, Sharmadean Reid's reach cannot be understated. Founder of boutique nail salon Wah Nails and community platform The Stack World, she's been challenging the traditional structures of beauty institutions since 2009 and shows no signs of stopping. Born and raised in Wolverhampton, Reid has become something of a London creative scene staple, facilitating and innovating how we navigate the world of business and figure out how to financially and

50

socially empower ourselves. Whether that's through our networks, investments, beauty, entrepreneurship or tech, Reid is constantly taking strides to expand the paths we Black women have been able to tread so far.

Naj Austin

Founder and CEO of wellness social club Ethel's Club and community audio platform Somewhere Good, Naj Austin is no stranger to a good idea. But her power doesn't just lie in the concept; it's also in the strength of her execution. Each of her business babies are unabashedly centered around community and people of colour. When Ethel's came on the scene in November of 2019 – inspired by and named after Naj's community-organising grandmother – it was one of the first of its kind: a subscription-based community space for people of colour.

Trinity Mouzon Wofford

As taglines go, 'a family business powered by 100% real superfoods' is about as wholesome as it gets. Founded by Trinity Mouzon Wofford, Golde is one of the most exciting sustainably-sourced wellness companies out there today – harnessing nature to create new, innovative ways to be well in our everyday lives. In an industry that is either overcomplicated by alienating language and impractical practices or diluted and simplified to the point of being ineffective,

Golde is a reliable, accessible platform that actually makes it easy, quick and even fun to take care of yourself.

Dr Mae Jemison

This last one is a name that I really believe we all should know. The living icon that is Dr Jemison was the first African American woman to enter space. Having been inspired by *Star Trek* and dreaming of becoming a scientist as a child, Jemison made the journey to space with NASA at the age of 36 as a science mission specialist – conducting experiments and research on the expedition. She had also served as a medical officer in the Peace Corps, she's a trained medical doctor and she runs a medical technology company. Can we hear it for The Woman in STEM?

WHAT DOES IT MEAN TO BE AT THE FOREFRONT?

There is a reason I wanted to highlight some key women in this chapter, and believe me, this list could have continued on and on. Choosing to centre Black women and our needs in conversations is crucial to changing the wider landscape of literally every industry. Whether it's women in science, tech, the arts, journalism or wellness, there is so much work to be done, and boy are there a lot of unbelievably inspiring women already getting their hands dirty. It's what this book is all about in a sense, but I think it's also important to acknowledge that it does come with its very own pressures and conflicts too. From bearing the brunt of emotional labour to double standards and the complications of success, it's not as easy as just shining a spotlight on ourselves and calling it a day. We are always facing the uphill challenge of fighting to be seen, to defy expectations, to deal with micro- and macro-aggressions, misogynoir, you name it. How do we overcome? Well, the first step is that we need to be armed with the language, the boundaries and the awareness to ensure that the change we push for is beneficial and sustainable in the long term, and we don't buckle under the responsibility of it all.

Black women have historically been at the forefront of change across politics and culture, fighting on behalf of marginalised movements worldwide, ranging from women's rights to civil rights to LGBTQIA+ rights. With so many of us sitting at the intersection of a number of these different groups, bearing the weight of that visibility constitutes a colossal amount of emotional labour. So often we are expected – or pressured – to do the work of making ourselves seen in societies that have been structured to erase us, forced to explain and justify our differences as if they are unnecessarily complex or other.

Even during times like June of 2020, when the world professed that it wanted to 'be seen to be listening and learning' in the wake of George Floyd's murder, the answer of who exactly was expected to be doing the 'telling and educating' was often automatically . . . Black women, of course. It's our job to challenge the status quo in the beauty world, to demand representation (in a palatable way), to speak up when something problematic occurs, to head up initiatives, launch businesses, advise the clueless and lazy and to mind our own personal experiences and trauma and project them on public platforms for brands, publications and our own social media in order to be seen to be giving enough. But where exactly does that leave us at the end of the day? Alongside many other things, it leaves our spirits exhausted and our souls depleted.

This is one of the many reasons why it's so important that in the process of bringing Black women to the forefront, we also bring forward concepts like 'emotional labour'. Sociologist Arlie Hochschild is the first recorded person to give a definition of the term, and while it's become pretty commonplace these days, it does bear breaking down. It's essentially the task of having to regulate your own natural emotions in order to fulfil some external task or play a role that is distinct from how you actually feel. In this case, it's the constant expectation of Black women to detach from their own feelings of hurt, anger and betrayal around injustices that they face, in order for us to embody the role of empathetic maternal educator and spirit guide instead. The real pain of emotional labour is in the fact that it requires a silencing of self, a repression that isn't healthy or conducive to healing or being well.

It can also become this breeding ground for other behaviours expected of Black women that are equally damaging. Like shrinking ourselves and our personalities generally to make others feel more 'comfortable' or less threatened or feeling like we have to assimilate and adopt the more common social language of spaces where we are the minority. It could also look like an internalised pressure to work 'twice as hard', to honour the old saying, or in Black spaces, could even look like a feeling of inadequacy around not being Black enough in the most immediate senses. You have to remember that while you are a Black Woman At The Forefront, you're not just any Black woman at the forefront – you're you. And that in itself is your superpower. You don't have to be anyone else or please anyone else or surprise anyone else even. You don't have to think of yourself as fighting for anything or falling victim to exceptionalism either. Just by virtue of being there and showing up as your truest self, you are doing exactly what you were meant to do.

In the world of being a Black woman, working, dating and families, as well as in some friendships, the truth is that being visible and having the mighty Black excellence trope thrusted on you can actually end up placing strain on those personal relationships too. Whether that's people feeling intimidated by the sheer size of your ambition or feeling second fiddle to it. This idea of 'having it all' in reality can feel a lot further away, and a lot of women in dominant professional positions can feel like they have to make a choice between their head and their heart. As that relates to a lot of our experiences as Black women, I think we also have this added layer of meaning that gets placed on top of our successes too, much like some of the names I mentioned above. Our wins are often cultural and historic too, ricocheting far beyond just the individual at the heart of them. While that's such a beautiful part of forging new paths, I feel like it can also end up skewing our priorities because we feel like our triumphs, even if they're painful or ill-suited to us, should come before our own wants and needs. That could look like taking that job promotion at a firm you're not happy at just because you know your parents and grandparents and uncle and aunt and family dog back home will be proud of you – because of what it *means* for your community. Or if you're in a public-facing field, that might be picking up gigs or commissions that don't feed your soul because you've looked and you're the only Black woman they reached out to, and you'll be damned if you give them an excuse to not represent us properly.

While it's true that *some* of these factors can definitely play a role in influencing the moves you make *some* of the time, we have to remember that at the end of the day our lives are really only our own to lead, and we can't allow ourselves to be ruled by these external influences to our own detriment. Finding the balance of letting your background and community guide and drive you forward, while also listening to your own intuition and desires is the only route to a long and rewarding journey at the forefront, I promise. If that looks like becoming a mother and taking some time off, that's what it looks like. If it's doing up career gworl, then so be it. There's no right or wrong way to succeed – you set the standard for yourself. I think it's what some of the women above do so well: they make their own rules, go at their own pace and set their own boundaries.

PRACTICAL COPING MECHANISMS

The burden placed on Black women by society – and even by ourselves – is immense, and finding ways to claw back control and creating peace for yourself under that kind of pressure always ends up feeling like an afterthought or a luxury you can't afford. Well, sis, I am here to tell you what you already know, and I will not rest until you believe it. Caring for others effectively and sustainably starts by caring for yourself. That's what this whole book is about: ways to be well for ourselves and also for the world. But when it comes to fighting for change, progress or success on the frontlines of whatever industry it is that you're in, making sure you're centred in your purpose consistently is at the very core of that. So, with that said, here are some of the best ways (big and small) in which I believe we can all get ourselves together.

Disclaimer: I am absolutely not reinventing the wheel here. There's a big chance you will have heard of some – or all – of these before, but if you're anything like me, when you heard these things recommended the first time, they might've sounded like bullshit. Five times later, and you're probably still not convinced. Ten times on, and *maybe* you've saved a couple tutorials on TikTok or IG but still no action. So, if I can be that *19th* time for even one of you reading this right now that pushes you to actually give some of these practices a go, I'll consider that a job well done.

First on the list is the idea of ROUTINE. To me, it always felt like a scary word because it felt like a polite way to say 'boring'. My instinct was that it was something to be resisted and avoided because it felt restrictive or predictable. But the older I got and the more the world threw at me, I started to realise that routine was actually one of the few things that could keep me grounded and sane in among the Wild Wild West of mental health, insecurities, changing jobs, friends, family, partners, etc., etc., etc. It's not so much about saying 'no' and being rigid or planning every minute of the day out meticulously. Instead, it's the small rituals and check-in points that you can give yourself that can prepare you for the war of everyday life and the beautiful and often scary unknown of everything else that we can't control.

The beauty of routines is definitely in their differences too. No two people's routines need to or should look exactly the same, in my opinion. The most important thing is to make sure that yours actually suits your needs and complements the way you want to live your life. If you love sleep and that makes you happy, maybe don't force yourself to get up at 5 a.m. every day because you saw one TikToker doing it and it didn't look as hard on screen as it feels IRL when that alarm starts belling off. We as a society have created these rules and the sense of morality around early birds being morally superior to night owls somehow, when time is, quite literally, a construct. Productivity doesn't always come easily to everyone so it shouldn't be at direct odds with your entire nature of being. Morning routines can be as simple as waking up, showering, brushing teeth, skincare, getting dressed and taking five minutes to make yourself the hot drink of your choice, then spending the 10 minutes it takes to drink it as quiet offline time before the craziness of the day begins. It could be leaving the house 10 minutes early to get that coffee from your favourite cafe en route to the station or picking a book or a podcast in advance of the week to fully enjoy on your commute. Taking those steps to find tiny pockets of joy and calm in the moments that we otherwise often go through on total autopilot can feel revolutionary when it feels like everything is expected of you once the day begins.

The same absolutely goes for nighttime routines too, as these moments can set us up to get the best rest possible and decompress. It could be playing white or brown noise sound effects before bed to allow you to fall asleep without the stressful sounds of tomorrow's to-do list clogging up your brainspace. Maybe it could be splurging on a nice little overnight lip mask that adds a bit of luxe to your bedside table following a YouTube scalp massage tutorial or it could even be taking that 10 minutes to moisturise your roots before bed but relishing the tenderness of caring for yourself in that moment instead of seeing it as a chore.

I read something really interesting about the science behind routine recently, too. And by 'read', I absolutely mean I saw a TikTok about it, thanks for asking. A neuro-scientist called Dr Chris Lee spoke about the reason that routines can have such a positive impact on how we navigate our day-to-day from the perspective of neuroscience. By creating these healthy patterns of behaviour and introducing more elements of what is predictable and known to us, we actively diminish the levels of stress or fight-or-flight hormones that spike in our body on a daily basis, helping us feel calmer, safer and more at ease in the long haul. I know that sounds really simple and obvious on a cultural level because we automatically associate routines with comfort and safety, but here's the little bit of trippy science behind it. Our central nervous systems literally look to our past experiences to figure out how to distribute our energy resources in future scenarios pretty much every second of every day, asking questions like 'have I encountered this before?', 'what happens when . . .?', 'does this mean that . . .?', and because of how we're wired, when we don't have the answer in our back catalogue of memories and experiences, our bodies naturally gravitate towards the worst-case scenario (because we'd always rather be overprepared than underprepared). So, when we build routines, we allow our bodies a level of understanding to know that because X has happened before, I know that X will happen next, aka everything will be fine, no need to worry. But when we live in these more consistently unstable states of being where our brains begin to believe that anything could happen at any given time, our bodies over-anticipate and burn through our energy sources way quicker as a result, leaving us simultaneously anxious and exhausted. It's probably the same reason you always feel completely knackered on holiday after just walking around in a new area or want to fall asleep at 7.15 p.m. when you've gotten back from your first days at a new job – your brain's in constant overdrive panic mode in its new surroundings. Even the smallest of routines help us fight against those instinctual anxiety patterns by building more certainty and healthy predictions into our daily lives, allowing us to function at a far more stable and positive capacity.

Another problem I always had with routines was that my own unrealistic expectations got in the way of me seeing them through. I'm sure you've heard this saying already, but people always tell you that it takes just three weeks to form a habit, and that's definitely a great benchmark to check in with yourself about whether what you're doing is working. The first week will feel the most unnatural but by week three, you hope that it's slightly less of a conscious effort. But it's also interesting to note that since that theory was published, other studies have come out suggesting it takes something more like two months before a new behaviour becomes anywhere near automatic. Which is a relief for me because it means I'm not broken. All I can say is, when it comes to building new routines, you have to account for bumps in the road too – it's not only natural but *expected* that there will be days when you don't want to follow your routine, when you just plain forget or when life happens and laughs at your plans.

I used to hold myself to a really impossible standard when it came to changing my life up, where I'd make super extreme shifts and then be surprised when three days later I'd already fallen off the wagon despite my best intentions. Nowadays I realise how much more value lies in imperfect consistency than in these all-or-nothing approaches. Don't beat yourself up for missing a week of journalling or gym or vitamins when your workload explodes unexpectedly; the world will absolutely keep turning. Just pick up the pen or the leggings or the capsule and try again.

Up second is MEDITATION. The best thing about meditation is that it comes in so many forms. It doesn't have to look like yoga pants in the lotus position with sound bowls. (Though I will say sound baths do actually feel like a massage for the brain, please go try one if you haven't!) But for so long we have been fed these super white-washed elitist ideals of who gets to 'indulge' in these practices and how much it should cost to do so. Spoiler alert: the answers are size eight white women in Lululemon, and a lot. But that's in pretty direct conflict with just about every tenet of Buddhism, and I also like to think that there's a distinction to be made between meditation in the strictest sense of training your mind to reach a point of total clarity and calmness and what I'll call meditative practices. The first I will leave to be taught to you by those with expertise. I really recommend the Calm app and The School of Life as starting points for beginning meditation, or even just taking time to go for a walk without listening to music and just taking in your surroundings and the sounds around you. Meditative practices don't necessarily require you to be sitting in a quiet room with your own thoughts, but this can make a really huge impact in helping you dull down the noise and cultivate a more positive mindset.

For some people cooking is meditative. The repetitive motions, the ASMR-as-hell sounds – it's an opportunity to tune out all the noise and give your mind some respite. It's also an inherently loving act to perform in nourishing yourself and your loved ones which equals bonus points. For some, running is meditation or painting or even cleaning. Whatever it is that you do where you find yourself able to still your thoughts and zone out in the best way possible can be a tool that you can use to practise mindfulness. There are so many incredible accounts across social media with easy-to-follow breathwork exercises or guided meditations that you can watch and learn to practise while you immerse yourself in a meditative activity. It's unbelievable how much the simple act of breathing and focusing on filling your lungs with air and your blood with oxygen for 20 minutes a day can shift your mood entirely.

Third on the list is JOURNALLING and/or GOAL-SETTING, depending on your own vibe. I really think that some people are just made for journalling and quite frankly, some are not. If you're the person at parties who can tell a story and have the entire room hooked on your every word or the friend who when you're in a fight with another friend or a partner is prone to blowing up people's phones with 'I just think it's funny how ...' paragraphs, followed by 'I'm sorry that ...' paragraphs, whether they've replied to the first one or not, journalling might be for you, babe! You need a place to channel all those feels. As a kid, I found the idea of writing in a journal so impossible. Which is ironic considering here I am literally writing a book at this very second. But something about the pressure of having to express myself so fully just made me clam up so badly; these days, though, I'm beyond jealous of people who get to look back at childhood entries and cringe out of their minds. I've just accepted that *me*, I'm better at planning and writing in list form instead. Way less intimidating for amateur writers and just as satisfying, despite what people say about writing lists being less productive.

If you're getting through it and it satisfies you, keep going. If it doesn't, that's a signal for change, sis – and that's on everything!

Whatever method works for you, I cannot emphasise enough the power of writing shit down. It sounds so simple but when you think about the number of thoughts and dreams and questions and worries that float around in our heads all day versus what we get the opportunity to share with those around us, it's kind of staggering the amount that gets left unsaid. Carving out time in your routine that feels realistic (could be daily, weekly, monthly) to sit with, organise and express what it is you are working towards, what you want and how you think you can get there, is an unbeatable way to not only clear valuable headspace but also start the journey of actualising your goals.

And outside of ambition-oriented writing, journals and list-making can be such an incredible way to practise gratitude and cure creative blocks too. One super-simple method I enjoy using is 10/10/10 lists, where you write three separate lists of 10. The first is a list of 10 things you desire in life right now, it could be career-related, health-wise, an actual object or activity, anything. Next you list 10 things that you are grateful for at this moment – think of a person in your life that you love or a memory you have or a situation you're in that you don't want to take for granted. Lastly, you list 10 things that you would really love to do – could be long-term goals, plans for the weekend or travelling or something that brings you joy that you just haven't done in a while. The idea is that it inspires you to recall the possibilities that lie ahead in your future, the things you have yet to do but have a passion for, and also reminds you of the things that you are already lucky enough to have today.

Fourth is MOVEMENT. I always feel like people say this, and for the first 95% of my life, my automatic response was to just roll my eyes. But post-pandemic, it seemed to just click for me. There wasn't one magical moment where I suddenly started to really enjoy running a 5K or something, but there came a time when I could just tell that my body needed to move. Whether it was a walk or a five-minute stretch on a yoga mat, there are some things that simply can't be thought through, they have to be felt and experienced physically. I think the easiest way to get into a rhythm of this, as with all things, is to just start small. Find the path of least resistance for you and make it as easy as possible to jump in and try to find a way to move every day, if you can. Something else that only occurred to me recently was that movement also doesn't need to be a chore or entirely serious to count. I can do a 20-minute Afrobeats dance routine on YouTube or pull up to the tennis courts at my park and hit a ball against a wall for half an hour, missing it at least 45% of the time. Embrace your time to move as an opportunity to switch off completely from your rational mind and just expel energy – be it nervous, frustrated or otherwise. Make yourself a little playlist or download a podcast, put the phone on Do Not Disturb and get in the zone.

Last, but by no means least, is THERAPY. I talk about it a lot throughout this book, so I won't over-egg the pudding now. In fact, take a shot (of ginger) every time I recommend going to therapy – your immune system will thank you. But in all seriousness, the simplest and

simultaneously most complex answer to dealing with all
that comes with being a Black woman at the forefront is
therapy. It's talking to someone, someone who knows what
to say back and whose job it is to do so. You may hear
'therapy' and immediately think, no way, too expensive!
But therapy doesn't always cost money – it can be obtained
through the NHS, support schemes and even through your
workplace. It's more accessible than you realise.

Four

BEING YOUR AUTHENTIC SELF

'Authentic' is one of those words that gets thrown around a lot these days. It does a lot of heavy lifting depending on the context. It used to mean everything from being unique or coming from a specific culture to describing someone who is truly down-to-earth and well-meaning, right alongside those who might self-label their own abrasive or straight-forward nature with it too. It's that thing that we all strive for and consider ourselves experts in spotting in others. It's a golden currency for brands and companies that want to connect with new audiences, and it's something that we take pride in when we feel like we can claim it. But what is the actual yardstick that we measure it with? How does a person achieve this kind of intangible quality? What even *is* it to be authentic?

In this chapter, I want to break the concept all the way down to its bones and examine how it manifests in our day-to-day relationships and what we often get wrong about it.

When I try to wrap my head around something that I'm struggling to understand, the first things I reach for as a starting point are usually definitions and examples. So first, when you look up the definition of 'authenticity', it's quite literally defined as 'the quality of being authentic', which . . . isn't exactly helpful. Dig a little deeper into what 'authentic' means and the gist becomes that it means something that's original, a genuine version of something, and if not the original then at least a convincing and accurate replica. For example, think about authentic cuisines. An Italian person who lives outside of Italy, or maybe even a non-Italian, could employ a recipe and their knowledge of Italian cuisine to create an *authentic* Italian dish without each ingredient having to emerge from the soils of Roma themselves.

When I apply that idea to humans and the way that we live, I think it makes total sense, then, that the definition of authenticity can differ vastly from person to person. There's no one way to be authentic. Often you see 'authenticity' thrown around and attached to a certain type of person or demeanour. Someone who #TellsItLikeItIs or who could genuinely pull off saying 'You can't handle the truth!' in the middle of an argument. Someone whose persona is 'real' and 'gritty', whatever that means. But that's literally not what authenticity means. If that isn't your natural way of being, what makes you happy or who you feel most comfortable being, then to strive for that is actually the definition of *in*authentic. Authenticity is about being the original and most genuine version of precisely who you are. It's not inherently authentic to only listen to Afrobeats and Highlife music because your parents originate from Ghana and anything else would be a betrayal of your culture and heritage. It's not inherently authentic to speak in one particular accent or wear one type of clothes because you have

68

a specific set of identities. It's authentic to do whatever it is that is true to your core, who you are and what you feel at any given moment. It's ever-changing and ever-flexible because it's not a description of one distinct characteristic – instead it's a description of the relationship between the way that you feel and the actions you take. So long as that link is real and as direct as it can be, then congratulations, because you, my friend, are living authentically as yourself.

Maybe it feels like I'm stating the obvious here. I'm aware that the statement I just made is absolutely easier said than done. 'Just do whatever you want, whenever you want!' she says. Sorted. No further questions. But that's not quite how it works in the real world. Society is so full of pressures and expectations and other humans with their other human feelings, thoughts and demands, and with bills that definitely do not pay themselves, what good is authenticity alone? In fact, valuing authenticity over everything and everyone else can end up sounding not just impractical but actually selfish when simplified to that extent. Sometimes you have to work a job that doesn't feed your soul to pay your bills, and you can't tell your boss precisely what you think of them. Or maybe the dream jacket that would represent you most is waaaay out of your budget for now. Practical life things are always in abundance, and to be honest, I think very very few of us are able to live a completely unobstructed life of authenticity, existing in a vacuum of our own realness. I'm not even sure what that would look like. Especially under late-stage capitalism. But at its core authenticity is really just finding and celebrating the parts of yourself that you wouldn't be whole without. And then making an effort to be conscious and feel empowered in the smaller ways in the everyday to pull out that truest self and give her room to breathe and stretch out in the world.

FOLLOW THE POCKETS OF JOY

So how do we actually find our authentic self? I hear you ask. Who is she? Where does she live? What's the best platform to reach out on? And unfortunately, there's no one right answer to this. Mainly because whoever your authentic self is, they're not this mythological entity like a fairy or a genie that exists separately from yourself and is sitting somewhere in a jar waiting to be unleashed with a magic spell. I kind of wish it was that easy though. Instead, your authentic self lives and breathes in everything you do, in the sparks of joy when you find things that you love and in the resistance and gut feelings of things that your spirit doesn't take to. Digging that self up and honouring it is a habitual practice of tuning into your intuition, detecting what makes you happiest and feeds your soul and finding ways to cling to those things and enlarge the portion of your life that they take up. That could take the shape of people, hobbies, career paths, food, lifestyle, your home, your daily schedule, your beauty routine. The beauty of authenticity is that it can be found and expressed in every inch of how we choose to live our lives.

We're all guilty of romanticising our lives a little bit, especially in the era of social media and constant documentation. But in this case, those obsessions can be super useful. Think critically about the moments in your life that stick out as the happiest. Ask yourself what it is about them that really felt joyous. Do any of them share commonalities? What are the running themes and how can you bring those into your life in an even bigger way? Notice your daily routines – when do you feel the most inspired and energised by what you have to do? What food makes you feel best? How much sleep? How much movement? When you're around people in your life, how do you feel? How do you show up? And crucially, how do you *feel* about the ways that you show up differently in different scenarios? I have certain friends that bring certain things out of me, as I think we all do. But I also go through seasons of enjoying and wanting to harness those different versions of myself, and not everyone around me is perfectly suited or compatible with each of those selves. And that's totally okay! In romantic situations or even familial, what kind of love do you want to receive? Are you communicating that with the people that need to know? Are you exuding that energy and taking the steps you can to make it possible? Are you playing an active and reciprocal role in this exchange and giving as much as you are taking, too?

These are all just some of the investigative questions I think we need to make room for in our lives on a regular basis so that we are constantly checking in on our own status on the path to authenticity.

THINK OUTSIDE THE BOX

There's no denying that we live in a society that really tries to tell us how to live: what's normal, what's good, what we should and shouldn't want to do and be. And some of the prescriptions it makes are totally valid. I like living in a world where we for the most part agree that murder is bad, just off the top of my head. Some rules exist for a reason, so that we can function (again for the most part). But other rules on the other hand, I think, are made to be broken. And that's why my next point in finding your most authentic self is just the recommendation to start thinking outside the box. Use your imagination when thinking about who you want to be. The options are quite literally limitless.

Now, depending on your background, your personality and how you grew up, every person's 'box' is bound to be different. If you grew up in a strict religious household, maybe pushing the boundaries for you looks like exploring your spirituality outside of that faith or watching *Lord of the Rings* because it was banned in your household as a child. For others, those boundaries could be different. It could be considering the rules of heteronormativity that have been imposed on us since we watched our first Disney film or moving to a different country and immersing ourselves in a different culture entirely. For model, speaker and the founder of Girls Will Be Boys, Char Ellesse, actualising her life as a Black queer woman and using her voice to speak truth to all of those communities is what she feels the most proud of. She says: 'When I started dating outside of cis men, it just felt like the missing piece of the puzzle . . . being a Black queer woman feels like I'm *complete*. I'm proud to be a part of all of those communities because they really feel like home.'

The unfamiliar and the unknown are naturally these slightly scary places for us, and we're conditioned to approach them with fear. But the more that you open your mind and ask new questions, sometimes the more you find new and revolutionary answers and new places to belong. So don't be afraid to push the boat out, whatever the boat looks like for you.

WHAT'S THE BEST THAT COULD HAPPEN?

At the same time, I'm not gonna lie, change *can* be extremely scary. And even when it's change that you want to happen, the next step of actually adjusting to it and explaining it to others can feel like its own special form of torture, too. On the most low-key scale, for example, when I worked in an office, as a Black woman, every time I changed up my hairstyle, I would dread going in the next day just because I didn't want to have all the conversations about how it grew so fast or whether it was really mine and how long it took to do. Sometimes you want a transition or a change to just feel seamless and like it's always been the case. You don't want to worry about questions like: what if they don't like it? What if it doesn't work out? What if it or I am just too much? In those situations, I've found the only way to reset my ever-panicking pessimist of a brain is to reframe my mindset completely. If our default is to consider and gravitate towards the worst-case scenario, I ask myself the question, what's the absolute best that could happen?

And when it comes to pursuing your authentic self via something you love, nine times out of the ten, the answer is going to be something undeniably positive. For example, there's an outfit that is a bit 'out there' and I'm scared about wearing it in public. What's the best that could happen? I put it on, I go out into the street, and I feel like an incredible new version of myself that I haven't before. You want to set up that IG account or website for the new creative venture you're scared to launch. What's the best that could happen? You realise it's what you're meant to be doing and it opens you up to new opportunities and connections that will help you thrive in the future. See where I'm going with this?

If you're still a little cynical, you can even practise this right alongside asking yourself what the worst that could happen is, too. Usually, the resulting answers to that question can help to remind you that some of the risks we take that we think are colossal like putting ourselves out there are actually quite small.

WELLNESS ACTION POINTS

1. Check in with yourself. Where are you right now in life – not in comparison to anyone else, but instead where you are, how you feel, how much energy you have at present, what energises you, what is taking your energy and what you honestly wish you could make more time for?

2. Write down three things you wish people knew about you. Then write down three steps that you're going to take to inch closer towards making these facts known to those close to you in the future. Maybe you've been routinely painted as the Strong Friend and people rely on you for emotional support, advice and strength, but in reality, you've just been afraid to be a burden in your friendships. Next time you're struggling with something or have a problem that needs solving, instead of freaking out internally and swallowing the stress alone, task yourself with confiding in one friend about what's happening. If it's that your love language is spending time together, but your partner has been communicating affection through gifts instead, make it your mission to let them know how much you love and value their company.

3. Watch yourself live a day in your life, and acknowledge and consider what could be kept, lost, improved upon and added. Take a notepad with you on a regular day and write down anything that you want to keep in your day (e.g. you have a project at work you are really enjoying), anything that you'd like to lose from your day that you do not enjoy (e.g. waking up late and rushing to catch the train), anything you think can be improved on (e.g. maybe you want to start listening to podcasts during your lunch hour) and anything you'd like to add to your day (e.g. spending more time with your

kid after work). This is a great way to learn more about yourself and to stop living life on autopilot.

4. Begin to identify and articulate the strengths specific to you. List them and try to add to this list on a weekly basis. Make this part of your routine.

5. Remember the last time you felt really good, full and proud of yourself. What talents were you exhibiting and what was the scenario? Save this and all the others on a Levelling Up vision board just for you. Bonus points for creating a digital version that you can access on the go – consider adding it to the 'favourites' file on your phones

6. Practise speaking as the best you – spoiler alert! She wouldn't be cancelling herself publicly at every conversational opportunity. Allow yourself to feel good and confident, to accept and bathe in a compliment. I promise you: you won't burst into flames.

Five

MENTAL HEALTH

There's a lot to unpack when it comes to Black mental health in the UK, USA and other parts of the Black diaspora. But unfortunately, when it comes to the information, statistics and articles out there, it seems like not many are up to the task. In fact, searching for tangible research and reports for the purpose of this book has opened my eyes to the fact that often in mental health, our problems and our questions can long go unanswered and without solution. In my own search, it left me with an unwavering feeling that no one actually cares.

Take the UK's healthcare system, for example. According to an NHS study* from way back in 2018, Black British women are significantly more prone than white women to experience common mental health problems such as anxiety, depression, panic and obsessive-compulsive disorders. In fact, less than 10 years ago, a government mental health and wellbeing survey showed Black women to be the demographic *most at risk* of experiencing common

---

* Department of Health & Social Care, The Women's Mental Health Taskforce, Final report, published 19 December 2018

mental disorders. Alongside this, we are disproportionately affected by the Mental Health Act at the same time.[*]

There's an understanding in the current medical industry that mental health issues in Black women are often dealt with during the more serious stages, as a result of delays in diagnosis, medical racism, historic cultural disparities in our understanding of mental health and also, frankly, a culture of Black women underplaying the gravity of their problems, or straight up refusing help if it is offered (instead hoping to save face) resulting in them seeking help for their issues much later in life or when the illness becomes severe. Left unattended to, these issues often present themselves as regular bouts of anxiety, fatigue, depression, lack of motivation (the inability to cook for ourselves, answer calls, respond to text messages), lack of emotion (empathy, compassion, social cues, positive and negative awareness), tiredness (i.e. simply getting out of bed, engaging in IRL social functions). Sound familiar? Well, yeah, me too, sis, and this is more widespread than any of us care to realise.

That said, Agnes Mwakatuma from the UK charity Black Minds Matter, and Real Talk Therapist Tasha Bailey both separately stated when interviewed for this book, that despite the concerns and red flags mentioned previously, the majority of individuals they are encountering who seek therapy and mental health assistance are Black women who have come to centre their focus, self-worth and identity in relation to their

---

[*] Refinery29, 'Black Women Are More Likely To Be Sectioned & I Have Been, Twice'

work personas. Let me land that one one more time. Even when seeking help or a route to 'get better', we are often seeing that as a path for our professional advancement rather than as an actual necessity for our own sense of wellbeing and happiness. The shackles of capitalism run *deep*.

It's a known fact that the Covid-19 pandemic in itself forced mass societal awareness around the challenges that have long-affected Black communities when it comes to the socio-economic inequalities we face both in and out of the workplace. Issues that were previously accepted as the norm or brushed under the carpet had room and momentum to surface themselves and demand discussion in the wake of us being disproportionately vulnerable, reckoning with blatant cases of injustice and state violence on a global scale or even just facing workplace anxieties and job insecurity at a higher rate than our counterparts. But no matter how much my Instagram feed and Twitter timeline tried its best to prove that the worst was over and change was afoot, I found myself continuously asking the question: 'is there anywhere on Earth that Black people are or can be safe?'

What about Black women? Where are we safe? Are we not even safe in our own minds?

When we hear Black women speak about having it twice as hard as everyone else, the world can often ridicule us or simply shut us down as overreacting, as if there's no proof. We just have to look at spaces like Sistah Space – a community-based non-profit initiative created to bridge the gap in services for domestic abuse survivors of African heritage – to get an idea of just how scary our lived experiences can be. But the truth is, in all our beauty,

'Any human can't be strong all the time, but I do think there is this extra pressure placed on Black women because of everything that we've gone through and all the generational stuff. We don't wanna let our people down as well because that's "our role" and we look at the strong Black women that came before us and think, I'm not doing enough, I need to be doing more. That's how I felt anyway, like I always needed to be doing more . . . That whole thing of "check in on your strong friend", who's checking in on the Strong Black Woman? Instead, we're left holding everyone up and then we're the ones that are burnt out.'

– Char Ellesse

our real and perceived strength, women from Black communities face the weight of both racial and gender inequality in pretty much every aspect of life, and that is bound to take a toll. Not only do we continuously take on the added responsibility of childrearing and childcare (single-parent and dual-parent households alike), but evidence provided by the Fawcett Society[*] explained that we are more likely than any other group to lose our jobs, to worry about debt and to be struggling in general to cope.

As I type this, I can almost hear my 73-year-old St Lucian grandmother saying consolingly, 'this too shall pass', like she always does. It's a saying like many others that a lot

---

[*] 'BAME women and Covid-19 – Research evidence', Fawcett Society

of us have probably heard growing up, and becoming all too used to it to ever question it, but the truth, and what we should all be asking in response, is: what if it doesn't? What then?

At some point we have to draw a line and stop adding to our load. We aren't superheroes or supernatural beings, we are humans with real feelings, emotions and limits, even if those are constantly pushed, expanded and invalidated. This all too well-known superhero complex that unwittingly resides in us all to some degree tells us that we not only can, but must, do it all and rest later or worse, 'when we're dead', as the saying goes. But in reality, none of this can wait. Our brains are mighty, yes, and we are strong, but being strong doesn't mean you're invincible, and that's something we need to learn to accept now if we are to build the infrastructures needed and constantly called out for in order for us to thrive, now and moving forward. If we want to begin to pass down a better future for our kids, to untangle and heal some of the generational trauma that has weighed down our families, it starts with us being our healthiest, happiest selves today. And we need room for that.

Support structures are few and far between. For those of us working and existing within the mental health and overarching wellbeing industry, this is not news. While our efforts aren't exactly wasted, they are without a doubt overstretched, and there's a valid criticism that there are nowhere near enough resources or funding to address the scale of varied issues that we're facing as a community right now.

The Mental Health Foundation concludes that due to the lack of adequate and sufficient data on Black people, they are most likely to be misdiagnosed, underdiagnosed and receive and have access to fewer treatments. Black women in particular have significantly lower treatment rates despite the fact that they are one of the most marginalised and disadvantaged groups in the UK, and as we discussed earlier, are often very acquainted with mental health issues on a personal level. Alongside this, there's a further lack of resources in terms of research and funding to find solutions to the crisis we find ourselves in, with the majority of work being done on a volunteer basis by charities and community organisations.

Speaking from a UK-specific lens, I personally believe that there is not enough coverage of the experiences Black women have when it comes to our mental health and medical wellness. While I could find books written from a more global diasporic perspective or even with an American focus in my searches, I came up pretty short trying to find anything to describe the distinct experience in the UK. One of the standouts however was an anthology edited by Dr Samara Linton and Rianna Walcott called *The Colour of Madness* that's just been re-released, which is well worth a read to further understand the experiences of Black and minority ethnic people in the UK.

As much as we are connected by our shared experiences across countries and continents, I do still believe that it's just as important to consider location and the nuances that come with it when discussing mental health too, from our cultural background to our socioeconomic standing in this country. It's also worth considering the generational gaps that mental health conversations bring to light. As Gen Z, millennials and Gen Y learn and shape the language of this new ground we're covering, the scepticism from baby boomers and beyond can be palpable. Mottos of resilience and coping, attitudes of insensitivity and entitlement – there is a habit of evoking the incomparable sufferings faced by those that came before us. But pain and oppression are not Olympic sports, there doesn't need to be a winner and a loser. And for us all to grow and exceed both our ancestors' and our own past selves, there's work to be done. Strength is an impressive trait, but it takes real courage to show vulnerability and to be honest about how we feel.

Resilience isn't a never-ending resource; it's only sustainable in the long term if we nurture it and know its boundaries in the here and now. Just because we have faced and overcome worse does not make today's challenges small or insignificant, and it certainly doesn't mean we can't try to change them. And ironically, once we've taken that step towards accepting change – which can already feel like a huge one – that's where the journey really starts.

You and I both know that we, as a people, like to talk. Lord knows we can talk till the cows come home. But sis, what is the use in all the talking – on social media, in our friendship groups, on panels, in speeches – if we don't take action? When speaking to community groups for the purpose of this book, the same issues came up over and over again. I ask leaders, what can we do? How can we make change? And they air the same frustrations. That not enough action happens outside of these conversations and that converts into the slow rise in our mental health problems as a demographic. Our intentions are well-meaning and pure, but often we, as human beings generally, are so put off when the results aren't as instantaneous as we want them to be.

There's that slightly cheesy and definitely overused saying, 'be the change you want to see in the world'. But in all honesty, I often think that when it comes to our health, we don't *see* ourselves as the change, we don't see ourselves as the main character in our own stories, instead we can be guilty of looking for someone else to save us. And unfortunately for us, the way the world's set up right now, often the people in those positions do not look like us or have a comprehensive understanding of our experiences as a demographic even. Far too often we resign ourselves to our suffering. Because we can't see the journey ahead of us or we think it's too hard, or maybe some messaging out there in the world has convinced us that it's what we deserve somehow. But I'm telling you right now, that though mental health explorations can be difficult and uncomfortable, and the road is not always entirely linear and not every day will be a resounding win, ultimately when it comes down to it, I can't think of a single scenario in my entire career where I've heard about someone *regretting trying to get better and investing in themselves.* So even when you're afraid or you feel like you're sliding backwards, try to remind yourself that you really do have nothing to lose in trying. And if you continue to choose you and push long and hard enough, there's actually a lot more that you stand to gain.

ADVICE

I am not a medical professional or a doctor and so you must not take my advice as gospel when it comes to mental health, however, I think it's important to share here the advice of professionals so you can gain some knowledge and understanding about your mental health.

If you are:
- worrying more than usual
- finding it hard to enjoy your life
- having thoughts and feelings that are difficult to cope with, which have an impact on your day-to-day life*

– you should consider seeking help from a professional.

If you are in a crisis and feel you have nowhere to turn, please call 999. It is never wrong to do this if you are desperate, and you will be supported immediately by healthcare professionals.

If you feel you want to look at different options to improve your mental health or resolve a mental health illness, then there are a variety of routes you could go down, including:

---

* 'Seeking help for a mental health problem: A guide to taking the first steps, making empowered decisions and getting the right support for you', mind.org.uk

85

- Texting 'SHOUT' to 85258 for an urgent NHS mental health helpline that is open 24/7.
- Booking an appointment with your GP.
- Speaking to a trained therapist.
- Reaching out and talking to trusted friends and family.
- Speaking to charities that can offer peer support, advocacy, crisis care and talking therapies.
- Seeking out workplace support – a lot of companies offer free access to support services through an Employee Assistance Programme.

For services that specifically serve our communities, I have made a list below that you can refer to whenever you need to. The people who run these spaces want to help you, and even if they are there simply for counsel and support, they may show you a route that really works for you that might be revelatory for your mental health.

BAATN – this is a site called the Black, African and Asian Therapy Network that enables you to find and contact therapists of colour, alongside free mental health resources.

Black Minds Matter UK – a network of Black British therapists that raises awareness about issues of Black mental health as well as providing resources and care for those who are unable to access them on their own.

Sistah Space – a community-based non-profit initiative

created to bridge the gap in services for domestic abuse survivors of African heritage.

Black LGBTQIA+ Therapy Fund – a fund system set up to help support those who exist at the intersection of the Black and LGBTQIA+ communities with access to therapy and mental healthcare.

Black Thrive – a south-London-based organisation run by those with social care experience to help support their local community.

BLAM – this stands for Black Learning and Mental Health and is a space and organisation dedicated to educating the next generation of young Black people on their culture, history and mental health.

Therapy for Black Girls – an online space and content platform devoted to encouraging the mental wellness of Black girls and women.

Celutions – an initiative founded to organise and create conversations around issues regarding Black mental health through physical and digital events and discussions.

Rainbow Noir – a peer-support and community action group that centres and platforms people of colour who are also part of the LGBTQIA+ community, both online and in person, mainly based in Greater Manchester and the north-west of England.

Six

GRIEF, LOSS & HEALING

'But what is grief, if not love persevering?'
– Vision in *WandaVision*

Something that we sadly deal with all too often within our community is loss. Whether it's the personal loss that happens within our families and friendship circles or the losses of our fellow Black people internationally at the hands of state violence, cruelty, war and corruption. When you think about what we've suffered through in all corners of the world in the past, it goes without saying that there's a further added layer of historic grief and healing that we all either have or will need to work through at some point in our lives. Studies into the impact of generational trauma are both totally shocking and yet unsurprising at the same time. A lot of the initial research into it was done in the sixties with a focus on the generations that followed Holocaust survivors. One study done in 1988 and published in the *Canadian Journal of Psychiatry* found that the grandchildren of Holocaust survivors were overrepresented in psychiatric care referrals by over 300%. The groups that scientists deem to be most at risk of similar emotional aftershock effects include those whose lineage has lived through years of war, catastrophes, abuse, poverty, racism and exploitation. Slavery, colonialism, anti-Blackness and all of the offshoots of violence and trauma that sprang from those systems fall squarely into those categories and make us susceptible to the effects of generational trauma. That trauma can then end up manifesting in any number of ways from anxiety to depression, mistrust, insomnia and can even affect one's immune system. Our bodies can literally be suffering through the pain and grief of our ancestors and our families as we speak, and we can simultaneously not even be aware of it.

If we want to interrogate every aspect of the lives we lead and figure out how to best cope and thrive on a journey towards wellness, I think exploring grief, loss and healing will form such key parts of that story as Black people and specifically as Black women, too. We often shoulder so much of the emotional labour and fight that comes with the more public and politicised losses, leading in organising and advocating for the rights of others over ourselves. In the homes where we are mothers, sisters, daughters, aunts and friends, when we experience personal losses, once again so much of that duty and responsibility can fall onto our plates both logistically in how we take care of those grieving around us and how we lead funeral preparations and also when it comes to the emotional heavy lifting. Running households, hosting guests, consoling, counselling, preparing, organising, maintaining some sense of normality amidst the chaos – all while trying to process and ground ourselves emotionally too. It's no surprise that many of us deal with burnout and straining mental health as a result.

Did you know that women are twice as likely to experience depression as men are, but Black women are *half* as likely to seek care or assistance with it?* I know we've already broken down the reasons why this can happen and how we can move forward, but I think that context is important when we think about the ways that we approach some of the toughest obstacles that life throws at us. Even if it hasn't happened for you yet, I can guarantee that grief has touched somebody close to you. And even though it's so universal and unavoidable, it still feels like this really taboo subject! It's everywhere, it's difficult and it's all-consuming, but we're all kind of too scared to talk about it.

Even when writing this book, this was the last chapter I started working on. It took me weeks to build up the courage to tackle it for some reason. To put it simply, I find it to be incredibly heavy and intimate. Ultimately, there isn't one circumstance of grief or one way to grieve. Sometimes we grieve communally, as we have seen on an international level, and then there is personal grief. Sadly, and sometimes frustratingly, there isn't a magical solution to deal with it. In most cases it requires a lot of time, space and perspective for you to feel like there's any hope at all.

While working on this book, I dealt with grief on many levels. I experienced the palpable loss of my uncle, the loss of romantic relationships and friendships and the loss of

---

* Johns Hopkins Medicine, 'Mental Health Among African American Women'

close family members that I had to remove from my life to repair painful parenting wounds. I have also grieved alongside and watched people close to me lose their parents, grandparents and friends, especially during the Covid-19 pandemic. I even experienced loss of myself and my dreams. The only way I can describe this season of my life in one word is: overwhelming. It's drained me professionally – stopping me from working on projects I have manifested and dreamt of for years, publicly and personally turning me into somewhat of a recluse as I've lacked the confidence and motivation to step outside and preventing me from holding conversations with people I know as well as those I admire. It knocked my belief systems: both my self-belief and my spiritual confirmation. I had become a fraction of the person I thought I knew, the person who believed so much in the vision of me running through my city and every corner of the internet spreading the hope and motivation I fought so hard to unlock. I lost so much, and there felt like no end to my grief, no solution. People who know or got to know me over this time definitely felt it, there was no hiding my unhappiness.

But what I did learn (eventually) is how to find light even in the darkest of moments and eternities because that's truly what it feels like sometimes. At times, I question who I continue to do it for, who I keep showing up for and why I force myself out of bed and into a routine. Do I do it for my son, my lover, my family, my friends, my community, the business, my clients and partners, to save face? No. I do it for me. I refuse to believe I was placed here and given these experiences for no reason. Without these painful parts of me, none of the magical parts would exist. That is my driver and I want you to embrace this belief too.

Yes, the world moves while and after devastating things happen but never in the same way. There is a humanity and an importance in each and every one of us in stepping back into and choosing ourselves when the worst happens. We are never alone in these experiences, and hopefully this chapter can provide some of the framework to understand the wider context of how we as a community deal with grief and also the tools to help you navigate through the storm of it.

OUR RITUALS

I think one of the most beautiful aspects of the diaspora that really hits home how vast and assorted we are is looking at the breadth of ways that we view and respond to the circles of life as communities. From the Caribbean to the regional traditions throughout the continent of Africa, all the way to the West, even in the moments of sharp, potent pain, we find ways to tell stories and locate the beauty within the darkness.

For many indigenous Black people and communities, death is a natural part of a spiritual journey: families and communities alike are known to uphold an open casket at funerals and to keep the remains of their deceased relatives in their homes for a number of days before they are eventually buried. Even then, they are regularly exhumed to be cleaned and cared for.

In the Caribbean tradition of Nine Night, this patiently stretched-out period of mourning spans, you guessed it, nine nights, culminating in a final celebration of the life of the deceased on the ninth night after their passing. In the days leading up, it's considered tradition to gather with those closest to the person who has passed and break bread over stories and memories shared fondly. It's this communal practice of processing and sitting with a new reality, all grounded in the belief that the soul of the person continues to linger throughout this time and oversee the proceedings in a way. On 'nine night', the last night, there's often a religious ceremony accompanied by hymns and prayer before the main gathering. The final occasion takes place in their house and serves as a send-off that liberates their spirit from its earthly ties and sets them free. There's usually music, dancing, storytelling, everything you might come to expect from a joyous event, sitting right alongside the heartbreak.

In my experience, and focusing on the St Lucian but very Westernised side of my heritage, I've seen a lot of changes to the Nine Night over the years. A lot of the practices depend on how senior and traditional the person who passes is. On these occasions, more formal customs prevail, like it being held in a house with elders and children separated room by room, a lot of talking and even exaggerated wailing outside from the immediate family (we all know that one auntie or uncle vying for attention) and zero music out of respect for the person who has passed. Whereas for my uncle's Nine Night, and others I have experienced in the last two years, there can be music, dancing, a hall hired throughout the duration, food catering and even a cutting down of the Nine Night to eight or even just one or two evenings. At the funerals, nowadays you see open caskets less and less, replaced with dress codes and themes usually honouring the deceased, drinking and pouring of good-good liquor onto the grave, less senior men from the community collecting money to top up the undertaker's pocket (bully for them), and something I am proud of experiencing, for the first time, is women being able to shovel the grounds over the lowered casket – a task that was almost exclusively held by men in the past. As you may have heard over the years from one mother to another mother's mouth, if the ancestors could see this they would surely 'turn in their graves' but the truth is, times are changing, and as we develop and grow as societies, it is natural that our customs will too.

It's actually said that elements of Nine Night may have roots within the religious traditions from across Africa too, some even stating that historically it was believed that when the souls were freed, they actually returned back to the continent rather than the generally accepted ideas of heaven that are the norm today. Of course, it would be pretty impossible to try and summarise all of the different death rituals that occur throughout the continent of Africa too, as many vary tribe to tribe before you even start to consider the differences between the countries. For example, when Nelson Mandela, who was from the Xhosa tribe in South Africa, passed away, he was buried in his home village of Qunu as a Xhosa chief. Some rituals were evoked to symbolise the return of his soul to his ancestral home, bringing his 'mortal remains' back so that there's harmony between the physical and the spiritual parts of him and they are tethered rather than disconnected from each other. In the case of Mandela, a senior person then performed a number of practices to help guide the spirit in its return to the ancestral home, narrating the journey back via the rivers and places crossed to get there, singing praise songs ('izibongo') from the person's family and lineage and evoking the names of ancestors that they will be united with. As part of the funeral proceedings, there's often a ritual sacrifice of an animal too called 'umkhapho' to honour their ancestors and aid the movement of the spirit through to the next world. The meat is then used to feed the mourners for the rest of the day. And when the mourning period ends, after a year, a similar practice called 'Ukuzila' happens to mark the end of it. A further ritual called 'Ukubuyisa' – which is said to bring the person back into the family as a guiding ancestor – may also occur. Like a lot of African cultures, there is a strong, unique connection to our ancestors just as there is a connection between the living and God or spirituality more generally too.

In Zulu culture, the deceased person is often buried with their belongings in order to aid their journey into the next realm. The Yoruba tribe often include things like food, clothes and other supplies in the burial. In Igbo traditions, it's preferred to bury those who have passed as quickly as possible to expedite their union with their ancestors, while in other tribes it's customary to wait for family to travel and arrive before doing so.

The first common theme that really stood out to me was the care and attention that we give to those we've lost even in death: providing for them, guiding them and doing everything we can to create the best possible foundation for the next chapter of their stories, whatever we might believe that to entail. Even in situations where we may not have access to the most resources, we find generosity and community to aid in how we honour the dead, and it feels like a selfless but also reciprocal act. Like an acknowledgement that we are as worthy and valued in both life and death. Another is the incorporation of celebration and joy. It is traditional in a lot of our cultures that the funeral will involve dancing and drinking and rejoicing. Celebrating the life lived and everything that person did in the time they had on Earth is just as important as recognising the loss. There is joy to be found in remembrance and commemoration, and our traditions have always allowed for this.

One of the other strongest threads I tend to notice across my limited knowledge and research of our elaborate diaspora is this important sense of homecoming in death which I think is incredible. This emphasis on us returning to where we began and to those who raised us here on Earth, but also a different but equal sense of homecoming in where we're going through our transition to the spiritual world too. Because so many of us have a concept of family and home that extends beyond the living to all those who came before us too, there's this reassurance that whatever happens next is not something you'll have to go through alone either. Whether you believe in a higher being or an afterlife, there's something so beautiful about the idea of there being someone waiting to welcome us on the other side, both as a person who is alive and as someone who's lost someone they love and wants them to be safe. It makes the path they're on seem like a natural and inevitable one, one that is less of an end and more another beginning. I'm sure, especially given the context of a lot of our ancestors, that this philosophy served as a great comfort for many and empowered them with the strength of an entire collective of people who are watching over them with love.

THE HEALING PROCESS

When it comes to those left behind after a devastating loss, it's a whole other story really, isn't it? Even when you're able to view the passing of someone you love as this beautiful journey and be grateful for what you had, the tough and painful emotions you go through when coming to terms with that are totally natural and human too and they can feel and become so intense that they threaten to swallow you up whole.

No one:
Black people: 'Good grief.'

Ever heard the phrase 'Good grief' and thought, *what the hell does that actually mean?* You're not alone. Black people sometimes say the oddest things during troubling times, and phrases like this used to make my nostrils flare and my eyes cut. Depending on who still says it, the vexing will continue to vex. But now that I'm on my wellness thing, I've been thinking about everything I was taught – the weird and downright confusing. So, is there such a thing as good grief? In short, yes. 'Good' grief has the power to unite families and even communities. If we open ourselves up to the opportunity, grief can help us grow and deepen relationships by enhancing our ability to grow in empathy and love for one another.

Something I've been working on for the last few years is to respect death and not be afraid of it. For as long as I remember I have been afraid of death, and I was never offered comfort or real understanding of what it meant. A fake-it-till-you-make-it mechanism of coping when it comes to death and grief is dangerous and is unsustainable. A lot of us hold

> 'Blessed are you who mourn, for you will be comforted.'
> – Matthew 5:4
> (paraphrased)

this fear, and it's completely natural and understandable, however it is often not helpful. Death is a natural part of life, and though it comes with a lot of pain, heartache and suffering, it is also accompanied by memory, love and an appreciation of the lives we lead.

To stop (or limit or control) my fear of death itself, I did the following:

- Realised that my fear of dying is actually stopping me from living.
- Engaged in actionable steps to become more comfortable with death. For example, by looking at statistics, reading books about death and its reverence with different societies around the world and reframing death in the view of 'a life well lived' or a transition.
- Talked about death more in vetted safe spaces.
- Created logical and positive affirmations and statements around death such as, 'it is as natural to die as it is to be born'.

Every single person's experience of death and their grieving process will of course be completely different, even when it comes to two people grieving the same person, so there's definitely no catch-all technique to overcoming loss. But even still, I hope that this list can at least serve as a resource of options to try to help you rationalise when the reality of death feels endless and scary and tiring. There are other things you can do too, and this chapter will guide you through them.

DON'T RUN FROM YOUR FEELINGS

When you're grieving, the sheer size of your emotions can often make it feel like the only way to cope is to run. The sadness and pain can feel so big and overwhelming that you can't even imagine ever being able to face it head on. Instead, the only way to continue to function is naturally to seek out all the possible distractions, pack the pain away and bury it under lock and key. And for a while, that approach will feel like it's working. You can get up and go to work and pretend things are fine, pushing down all the flashes and reminders that hurt too much to look at. But sometimes I find that the less attention you give the pain, the more it can actually start to bubble up and grow exponentially, until it reaches a point that it's so big you have no choice but to pay attention to it. It'll grind you to a halt in the shape of burnout, breakdown, illness, undirected rage or any other number of ways.

I know it sounds easier than it is but my first tip for coping is to force yourself not to run from your feelings. Grief is entirely natural, entirely valid and an entirely necessary part of loss and of life in general. It's not something you need to feel ashamed or scared of. Instead, the only way to slowly but surely decrease its sting and find ways to live and move forward with it is to give ourselves the time and opportunity to fully come to terms with all of its nooks and crannies. To stare it in the face and sit with it. In the more immediate sense, that might look like granting yourself the grace to really let your emotions out instead of fighting them back. Crying it out, screaming it out, practising stillness, honouring solitude when you need it and asking for help and to be held when that's what your spirit is calling for. It's a process of open communication within yourself and with those around you who love you and are here to guide you through the storm too. Even if you change your mind, even if you contradict, even if there's no magic button to fix it.

Another thing to remember is that the emotions you feel are not always going to be entirely straightforward either. Sadness is not the only valid emotion of grief. You might feel angry, you might feel numb, you might feel betrayed. Our lives, relationships and emotions are messy, so naturally our grief surrounding them will be too. Adopting a mindful approach to how we attend to our feelings in grief stops us from suppressing the feelings that we don't think we should be 'allowed' to feel. That could just be giving voice to them as they flicker through you, writing them down in a journal, a letter, speaking them through with a friend you trust or a therapist – not giving them power over you by trying to control how they manifest or keeping them hidden.

THERE'S NO TIMEFRAME

This is something that you hear a lot, but in practice it can still feel hard to remember. Grief is something that we imagine ourselves pushing through and emerging out on the other side of, but in reality, it's something a lot less linear and a lot more complex than that. Another part of healing might look like acknowledging what has happened and how it has and will continue to change you. The pace of your life before and after loss do not need to match up, the things that you enjoy might not be the same and new things might trigger you. Though their rituals may have set timeframes in traditional settings, grief and mourning aren't confined to finite periods. Two weeks off work won't cure you of it. There really is no timeframe for healing and healing in itself doesn't even necessarily mean that the loss will never hurt again. More often than not, healing from grief doesn't look like the grief disappearing from your life, but more like the rest of your life and you growing around it and through it.

My advice is to just be as patient as you possibly can be with yourself, because to be honest, there probably won't be one clear day when you wake up and suddenly feel significantly better like you've gotten through the worst of it. At the same time, you may have a day that feels like that, and then a month later, something happens that brings you all the way back down and it feels like you've lost 'progress'. But we can't necessarily think of grieving as working towards this eventual glorious end goal of no more pain. It will come in waves and bursts that you both can and can't explain sometimes, and just because it still hurts doesn't mean you're failing or stuck.

GROUND YOURSELF

Often when people talk about even the first moments of losing someone, there's a language of feeling untethered or weightless as the news flips your entire world upside down. While it's not always possible to do so right away, as time goes on, it's crucial to find ways to ground yourself and connect with your surroundings in grief as a way to help you feel less lost and alone in it, and to remind you of the beauty of what you do have and what has not been lost too.

I know it sounds super clichéd, but nature really is a great way to start that process and that can look as big or small as you feel ready for it to. It could start with buying yourself one small plant and challenging yourself to water it once a week (maybe a succulent as those pups are real sturdy even if you forget), or it could be taking a 10-minute walk and sitting in your local park just taking in some fresh air. If you have the opportunity to get away, a spiritual retreat somewhere with water and trees could create a really incredible healing space for you. Just finding opportunities to relate to something outside of yourself again like your environment can help bring you back down to Earth.

Once you're in the habit of that, I'd also highly recommend breathwork and/or meditation as an additional layer to grounding yourself in nature. Even if it's just as an exercise to breathe more deeply and get more oxygen into your system if your brain feels too busy or fuzzy. It can be something to focus your energy on to stop your brain from wandering and allow you to feel fully present in that moment at least.

DON'T BE AFRAID TO REMEMBER

I think often, much like the first point, we can end up believing that the only way to heal fully is to suppress – whether that's emotions, memories, even just talking about the people we've lost. There can be this idea that if you talk about something often, it means you haven't healed from it. But I don't think that's true.

Someone close to me once described how they knew they had started to heal as the moment when they were able to remember certain stories or moments with the person they lost, and instead of the memory making them feel empty and hurt inside, they were able to find joy and peace with it again. The wound wasn't reopened; it had healed over in a way that meant the memory of the person was no longer shrouded in pain. I found that a really beautiful barometer of grief as something that doesn't necessarily disappear but just lessens in its dominance of all your other emotions including those evoked through memory.

I think grief can often feel like it robs you of your connection to someone for that exact reason. You're scared to think of them, to be reminded of them, because the pain is too much to bear. But once you push past the most raw and emotional weeks or months of grief, there is a barrier to be broken and braced through in order to reclaim your love for that person as something that doesn't just hurt you anymore. It can be full and complex and, of course, still painful, but also joyful and comforting too. It can still hold all of the beauty of the relationship you had before your loss; it just takes a minute and some perseverance to get there. To get used to speaking and thinking about them again, laughing at your funny stories with them, looking at pictures and videos. But ultimately, it's one of the best ways to hold on to them and honour their personhood and legacy too. So, this is your reminder to not be afraid to start remembering again when the time is right. To spend time in nostalgia and immerse yourself in all the things that you loved in them again, remembering that they can continue to bring you joy and peace on your journey through the experiences you already had and that those live on through you and your memories of them.

HOW TO SUPPORT SOMEONE YOU KNOW IS GRIEVING

1. The first thing to do is reach out. Don't wait. Be open. Something like 'I'm here if you want to talk' or 'Is there anything I can do?' is good. Judge their reaction and base your support around this.
2. Try not to rationalise the death or the situation. Phrases like 'everything happens for a reason' or 'things will get better' are often unhelpful and can be frustrating to someone in the midst of grief.

It may feel like you can never get it right, but the most important thing to do is to be present for when that person or persons need you.

3. Be available to listen to them and ensure that boundaries are discussed for both sides so each person feels protected.

4. Sometimes physical contact or an act of service is all that's needed. Ask if they need a hug, a babysitter, company to arrangements or meetings or if you can make them a few dinners that they can put in the freezer.

5. Understand there will be good days and bad days. Don't judge them. Be their stability and a constant. In times of grief everything can feel up in the air; knowing they have you is a reminder of life's routine and resilience.

Loss is an inevitability, and it's something that connects us all as humans. It allows us to relate and to come together and it can promote great bonding between us. None of us are alone in our experiences. And who knows? A loss may open a door to new love and new connection.

Seven

BLACK BEAUTY

'To be an active space for the celebration of Black beauty, and for authentic beauty, and to let ourselves be the subjects of our content.'

— Tracee Ellis Ross

HOW DO WE DEFINE BLACK BEAUTY?

And now, we arrive at the subject of Black beauty. And no, I'm not talking about the famous horse. I mean the colossal, complex industry, lifestyle and culture that forms a huge part of everyday life for a lot of Black women and Black people in general. I'm glad to say that it's a term filled with a lot of joy and richness today, but it also carries a lot of weight and history in a world that has often attempted to erase it, question it and shape it. Each of us has probably been on a journey to unpick what our own relationship is to Black beauty outside of what the world tells us it should be, but no matter what stage of that journey you're at, here I want to dig into some of the main areas that make up this huge part of our lives and why understanding them and thinking about them critically is so integral to how we take care of ourselves and progress on our path to being well.

Before we dive into the world of beauty as it pertains to Black women and people, I figured it'd make sense to acknowledge some of the debates about beauty versus wellness too and where I stand on them. There are some schools of thought that make a really clear distinction between where beauty ends and wellness begins, while others see their boundaries as far more fluid than that.

Generally, when we talk about beauty, we're thinking about practices, tools and products that are concerned with our aesthetics, aka how we look on the outside. That would include areas like make-up, hair, cosmetic surgeries, and maybe even things like our nails and our skin. Of course, beauty is something that exists in the world around us as well – in nature, family, friendship – but in this chapter, we'll just be looking at it as it relates to us and how we look and are perceived. While it's super valid to argue that these rituals sit separate to our wellbeing, if wellbeing is defined as being healthy and improving our internal qualities, I think it's beyond important to understand the links between our wellness generally and how it manifests through our relationship with beauty. Do we wear our hair a certain way because we like it and it's practical or because we have some buried prejudice about what 'good hair' needs to look like? Why do we never leave the house without our hair 'done' or make-up covering our skin? Would we feel comfortable if we did? Are the standards we hold ourselves to there to benefit us or to restrict us?

There's no right or wrong answer either when it comes

to this, it's not that if you reach a level of peak internal wellness then you automatically no longer see the appeal of make-up and other cosmetic processes, nor is it the other way round either. Placing value and time into your beauty routines isn't inherently a symptom of not loving yourself fully. For each person, that relationship will look totally different and the reasonings behind your actions are just as, if not more, important as the actual act itself.

Not only that but it's been pretty universally acknowledged that in other ways, taking care of our physical and emotional health also means that we are able to look at ourselves through a more positive lens, and taking care of ourselves physically can provide a much-needed confidence and energy boost when you're feeling down. You know that feeling you get when you haven't worn make-up for a while, and you get your full-face beat on and forget how to act? Or when you've got a fresh set of nails on and it feels like a joyful little piece of armour that makes you ready to face the world as your fullest self? Sometimes the power of beauty is purely in the decision to take that time for yourself and pour into the things that make you happy, even if they don't feel as important as the deeper work.

The reverse of this is that we all have a lot of work to do to interrogate our motivations for partaking in various beauty practices to ensure that we don't become too reliant on them or use them as a means to distract from or further worsen our deepest insecurities. We have to consider our actions fully to see if there is something going on behind them. For example, are you spending more money than you can afford on beauty treatments as that is the only thing that makes you feel better about yourself? Or do you feel lesser than because your body doesn't suit the outfits that look perfect on slim models? It's key to assess what we are doing and consider if our actions are due to societal or external pressures or if they are unhealthy coping mechanisms. To acknowledge our vulnerabilities is a strength and when we acknowledge them, we can usually see if our actions are actually benefiting us and improving our lives or if they are making things worse.

With social media today, we are ingesting so many subliminal messages through the images we consume that whisper doubts and unattainable standards into our subconscious, which can take control of us without us even noticing. We are fed images of a standard of beauty out of our reach and made to feel we have to match up to other people's highlight reels and edited versions of themselves. It's not an easy world to navigate. But being able to pick ourselves and our own goals apart from what we're being told to think and value is something that can only come with experimentation and self-reflection because the answer is often buried deep under excuses and justifications, as well as being perpetuated by a society that absolutely does not care if we do the work or not, as long as we're still spending the coin, sis.

BLACK HAIR

Black women's relationship with our hair is so often formative. Whether you grew up having it relaxed, straightened, tucked away in braids or it was left to do its own thing, we all have a hair journey that may have taught us how to relate to our Blackness and our perception of beauty from an early age.

It's up for debate whether our hair is inherently political, with compelling arguments on both sides. Some bring up the inherent symbolism of the Afro during the civil rights movement as a beacon of embracing our Blackness in the face of oppression. They believe that Black hair in its natural state is a form of resistance – especially in a world that deems it 'unruly', unprofessional or as some kind of beast that needs to be tamed – and for many, learning to love and appreciate their hair in its natural form really is a radical act. When you read the work of academics such as Emma Dabiri, author of *Don't Touch My Hair*, you get a sense of just how deep the revolutionary nature of Black hair goes back in history. From braiding patterns used to hide grains of rice and seeds during the Middle Passage through to patterns linking back to some of the earliest forms of mathematics, Black hair is so rich in history and subtext. At the same time though, others will insist it really isn't that deep, or at least that it shouldn't be! The fact that our hair has even become a topic of debate and contention is restrictive in and of itself, and it's only when our hair is seen as precisely what it is (i.e. follicles that grow from our scalp incidentally) that we will *truly* be free to do what we want with it. Not every choice we make has to have some deeper meaning. Taking it further, they might even add that the decision of a person to keep their hair natural or not shouldn't be imbued with some deeper moral notion. Whether you opt to weave your hair, cover with wigs, loc it, braid it or shave it all off, that decision should lie with you and you alone and doesn't need to communicate a broader truth about who you are and how you see the world. Whichever camp you fall into though, I think we can all agree that the discussion alone and the beliefs held around Black hair and its significance, show just how nuanced and central it is to our idea of self, wellness and also our participation in our community too – from sharing tips, having the hard conversations, to your relationship with your own braiding ladies, it's something that binds us together.

When it comes to the natural hair movement, it's hard to know where to start. It's ever-changing and has enriched so many of our lives as we teach and learn the best ways to relate to our hair. Though there are probably about a million and one different schools of thought on the order in which to moisturise your locks alone, it really does feel like so much of the communal natural hair journey we get to see expanding in real time is like watching history in the making. To think that we have probably never known more about what our hair needs to thrive than we do right now and that there is still so much to come is so beautiful and exciting to me.

At the same time, like most movements it has its blind spots. Texturism is still a huge problem when it comes to who is platformed as the face of the movement and given the space to speak. Showcasing and understanding the vast range of hair types we have under the umbrella is precisely what makes Black hair so impressive and rich, but at the same time, we have to be hypercritical when spotting the patterns of which ones are pushed to the forefront and awarded visibility. And it's not just an issue because representation is a 'nice to have', but because the needs and experiences of different hair textures are fundamentally different and so lead to different lived experiences. Those with looser curl patterns should not and cannot speak on behalf of those with coiled hair and vice versa. When it comes to the challenges and prejudices faced out in the world or even at home on wash day, even if our definition of 'good hair' has expanded to include some kind of curly patterns, we haven't reached the point yet where all curl patterns are viewed as equal.

One exercise that I found really helpful in my own journey with my hair was taking the time to learn it and enjoy all of its behaviours, rather than trying to bend them to my will, fight them or just straight up work against them. My hair isn't always going to do what society has told me it is normal to do. When it grows, it won't do that straight downwards, when it's wet, it won't get straighter, when I comb it, it won't alway look 'neater'. But when you stop viewing those differences as a downside or ways that your hair is falling short of the norms or making your life more difficult, you start to realise they can become superpowers. During lockdown, I would set myself the goal of keeping my hair out and natural for an elongated period of time and then allowing myself to experiment and play with it without the pressure of time commitments or having somewhere I needed to be – the things that often force us into a pattern of frustration, stress and attempts to look 'presentable', whatever that means. Instead, that opportunity to engage in no-strings-attached play mode genuinely felt like reigniting something within my inner child who spent hours sat between the legs of aunties wrestling to 'tame' and primp me into acceptable shapes as I writhed and whinged. After some sweary mirror sessions, a few questionably loose 'dos and days of achy arms from contorting myself to reach the back of my scalp, the magic of the coil felt so much clearer to me. My hair took on this quality as something that was more alive and autonomous, that needed to be nurtured back to health so that it could bounce and curl and thrive, rather than this inanimate object to be projected on and subjected to my every whim. Instead of wanting to work against my hair and dampen its nature, I found myself gravitating towards all the things you're told not to do too much with your hair – wetting my curls to see them regain their shape, leaving my edges loose, flipping all the standards that I never even got the chance to consent to in the first place. The more I explored, the less tied I felt to these rules and regulations I had assumed I needed to follow in order to feel beautiful, and ironically, my hair was happier than it had ever been. It grew more in the time I was staying my ass in the house and doing whatever I wanted to it than it had in any other set of years combined in the 'protective' styles I had been too afraid to stray from.

I say all that to say that I relate *hard* to the fear and frustration that can come with getting to know our hair. It can feel unfair that alongside everything else we have to deal with, here's one more skill we have to master just in order to live. We have to be sisters, mothers, wives, therapists and now hairdressers too. But our hair is a part of our body, our vessel, and the more we learn to be in harmony with it and learn what works for us, the more in tune with ourselves we feel too. And that doesn't need to be a high-maintenance routine either. Like any other body part, it's just about seeing it for what it is, accepting it as such and figuring out how to make it work best for *you* and the life you lead. That could be switching up styles every week or shaving it off completely. It's your body, it shouldn't be holding you hostage.

I'd also like to take this opportunity to remind you that all the rules we tell ourselves about our hair, that we judge ourselves and others on? Plot twist: they're literally all made up. Your edges don't need to be laid, your hair doesn't need to be a certain length before you can wear it down, your curls don't need to be a 3b texture for you to rock an Afro, your ponytail doesn't need to be rock solid for you to be seen as a baddie, wearing a wig doesn't mean you don't love your natural hair. Too often we as Black women can start to internalise the scrutiny that we're put under to be immaculate at all times in order to be deemed worthy. That needs to end like yesterday. The beauty in your hair lies in its connection to the beautiful *you*. And if you want to rock whatever style you want to rock, a) it doesn't always need to be perfect and b) you should do it because it makes you happy, not because you're worried what someone else might say or think about you.

Top hair tips:

- Always sleep with either a bonnet or a scarf to protect your hair and so it doesn't become rough.
- Watch YouTube videos of Black women with the same hair texture as you to discover different ways of doing your hair – the knowledge they are sharing is free and often extremely helpful!
- Take baby steps – you don't have to try everything at once.

BLACK SKIN

According to our good sis Solange in 'Almeda', Black skin is a luxury in and of itself. We hear it talked about that way all the time, in poetry, in music, in literature. From the beautiful breadth of shades it comes in to its propensity to 'not crack', as they say, our melanin is not something we should ever take for granted – no matter what comes with it. Despite its magical qualities, however, and outside of the cultural institution that is cocoa butter, it hasn't always been the case that we really know how to take care of the skin we have in the best way possible, sadly. Myths about not needing to wear sunscreen or misinformation about what certain skin conditions look like on us are a result of a lack of representation within dermatological research rooms and labs, and to be frank there's also a historical lack of access and time to spend digging into the education out there about these things too (we've had quite a lot of other shit going on as a people, I don't know if you heard). But something that I think is really exciting about this new age of skincare is that we are learning so much about the deep science and workings behind the products we use and the requirements to keep our skin looking as good as it does right now. Instead of just trusting what's on the bottle – the marketing ploys and language used to convince you that you've found the silver bullet – companies and individuals are peeling back the curtain to break down how skin truly works, what it needs and where to go to find it across a range of price points. With regards to Black skin, in particular, it's been a long time coming.

Like with most industries, Black women are and have historically been viewed as a slightly irrelevant minority when it comes to skincare. And while many of the myths have already been debunked around the ways that Black skin might be different to non-Black skin (I will say it again, yes, you need SPF), there are still some ways in which our skin is different and requires specific awareness.

Dr Hani Hassan is someone who's been super vocal in this space and made it her mission to demolish the jargon and gatekeeping around dermatology with a specific focus on areas of particular concern for us melanated folks, for example, hyperpigmentation or skin bleaching. Her Twitter profile and YouTube channel are wildly informative on these subjects that can often feel like a bunch of excessively long, made-up words that all kind of sound the same. She breaks down recommended skincare routines, ingredients to look out for and be wary of as well as the causes behind some of the skin concerns that disproportionately affect us. Another great voice in this space is Monique Monrowe aka the Skinfil-trator, an aesthetician who has taken to TikTok to educate the masses on everything from skin barriers to waxing. She provides product reviews and how-to guides alongside speaking directly to a melanated audience about the topics that affect us most. There are definitely so many more out there doing the work too, but those are just two examples of Black women who are taking steps to make skincare knowledge accessible and universal, something that we unfortunately often have to do for ourselves because the myths run deep.

As we've seen, it's pretty much impossible to talk about Black beauty without talking about the role that Eurocentrism, colonialism and racism play in corrupting our perception of it. Especially when we think about Black beauty as it's perceived in the global West, although the reaches of it can very much be felt throughout the diaspora with practices such as bleaching and lightening, too. To this day, it's disappointing to still hear horror stories of products still being made that are harmful and damaging for melanated skin. Meagan Good recently spoke out about being prescribed a skin cream that contained bleaching agents and not realising until it was too late. The product was meant to treat sun damage but ended up lightening her complexion notably, to the point where there was speculation online. When she addressed the rumours, she even commented in an interview: 'It broke my heart to think that there's little girls seeing this commentary and thinking it's true.'

Recently, someone I know had a similar experience after going to a specialist for her own skin concerns. Despite repeatedly asking the doctor if the product was a skin lightener and explaining that she didn't want that, she was prescribed a product that started to exhibit lightening symptoms and she immediately stopped use. But by that time, some impact had already been made. Luckily, in both of these cases, the results have not been permanent but it's a really frustrating example of how even presumed specialists that we are meant to place our trust in are *severely* lacking – if not negligent – when it comes to knowledge on Black skin. In this big 2022. This is my plea to all of us who are embarking on our skincare journeys to take even a couple of hours to watch a few short videos on how to best take care of your skin and what to look out for before buying new products that are marketed as a quick fix for all, because often that all doesn't *actually* mean to include us. And as we fight to unlearn our own internalised prejudices and embrace our skin, we still have to be super wary and conscious that the set-up out there in the world is still primed to work against that.

Top skin tips:

- Don't overcomplicate your skincare routine. A good cleanser, toner and moisturiser are all you really need to keep your skin healthy and happy.
- Niacinamide or using retinoids can be great to reduce pigmentation and even out your skin tone.
- Don't sniff at a good Lidl serum – if you just need some hydration, it does the job!

PLASTIC SURGERY

You knew it was coming, and we have to talk about it. Plastic surgery is an ever-growing phenomenon, both in the beauty world and in the 'real world'. Whether consciously or subconsciously, it will impact every single one of us at some point or another. In 2021 and in the UK alone, roughly 15,000 cosmetic procedures were performed. From smaller tweakments such as filler and botox to more invasive procedures like BBL (Brazilian Bum Lift) and breast enlargement, it's clear that the accessibility of plastic surgery is growing. According to the British Association of Aesthetic Plastic Surgeons' statistics, 93% of cosmetic procedures performed in 2021 were on women.[*]

Women are altering, adjusting and changing their bodies at an exponential rate, and the movement is showing no signs of stopping. When you are scrolling through your Instagram and TikTok feeds, it's highly likely a considerable proportion of the people you are seeing have had 'work' done. This feeds into the inaccessible beauty standard that can make you feel like you're not good enough: your breasts aren't big enough, your waist isn't small enough and your bum isn't giving shelf enough. As Black women especially, we feel so much pressure to look pristine and perfect to feel beautiful, in a world when so many (lucrative) systems tell us we're not. Plastic surgery is an attractive thing as it can make us feel like we can fix everything with one prick of a needle or swipe of a knife. But it's so important we take a step back and assess what surgery really means on a deeper level, and in a wider context. It's also incredibly important that we really do our research before jumping into the deep end of an industry we know very little about as untrained medical participants. We need to be aware of the very real effects on our physical and mental capacities both before and after treatment and to make sure we are aware of the aftercare, which hardly anyone speaks about. It's also key, before we

---

[*] Analysis of BAAPS Audit 2020–2021, Baaps.co.uk

embark on this, we understand how unrealistic it is for all faces, bums, tums, arms, boobs, legs and all the rest to look a) perfect and b) the same as everyone else's. Your unique features are steeped in history you should really be proud of – many haven't made it here and your body and face are temples. They are beautiful as they are.

That said, I am very aware of the movements for and against non-surgical and surgical cosmetic surgery. In the 'for' camp, a lot of women will say that getting surgery is a form of empowerment and a new kind of feminism. Listen, I get it. Taking control over your beauty and throwing aside those insecurities can probably feel like empowerment in the moment and we all want to feel good about ourselves and have confidence. But will it really resolve all the deep-rooted unhappiness within you to look in some way, shape or form like people you don't actually know who are influencing you in ways you aren't completely aware of? And at what cost does this action come to you health, your loved ones and the wider community? Ultimately, I feel that everyone should have the freedom to do what they feel is right for them, and I will never hold any judgement for people who decide to have surgery. Some people get surgery to resolve trauma, others as gender affirmation and some invest in it to further their careers. The number of different reasons women in particular go down this route are vast and valid. However, I think to not criticise the industry and to paint it all over as something that empowers women and that is a positive force for good is dangerous and not nuanced enough.

Women, especially Black women, are working against

a system that aims to invalidate them and make them feel like they are missing something so that they invest *money* into changing that. A patriarchal system wants us to be visually pleasing to them, a white-supremacist system favours women who look a certain kind of way and those who are closest to a 'whiteness' in features, and a capitalist system wants us to spend a lot of dollar. And when I say dollar, I mean a *lot* of dollar. Some of these procedures are *expensive*, and if you can't afford to buy it twice, you shouldn't buy it. It's not worth putting yourself in debt, as you will be creating another problem for yourself in doing so. Shout out to you, depression! Alongside the cost of these procedures, we also need to consider the health risk. We can't forget or simply ignore that Black women do experience less than adequate care from healthcare systems in general. It's a fact. Embarking on a procedure, any procedure in fact, puts you at risk of experiencing medical racism, negligence and even results that could be life-threatening and frankly irreversible. Due to the high cost of these procedures, often women look to get them done in other countries (such as Turkey or Brazil) and this can come at greater risk. In fact, in 2022, there has been a 44% increase in botched procedures from abroad, according to BAAPS and *The Harley Street Journal*.*

These practices are becoming normalised and more widely accessible, but this doesn't mean they are good for us or should be embarked upon lightly. They are not a

---

* *The Harley Street Journal*, https://theharleystreetjournal. co.uk/2022/04/25/

quick fix for a long-term, deep-rooted insecurity or mental health problems, and they are often permanent and can be lifechanging. Is it an enhancement or a devaluing of who we naturally are? I can't say for certain. I just think, as in everything, it's all about balance and being self-aware and self-critical. If you are considering plastic surgery, whether it's lip filler, a tummy tuck or breast augmentation, take the time to really think about it. Write down your reasons why and your reasons why not. Other methods, such as mindfulness and wellness, exercising and moving your body, and self-confidence workshops, are alternative ways you might be able to resolve or embrace what you want to change. Think about the bigger picture: imagine a teenage girl following you on Instagram who is so happy to see you have a nose like hers and that you love yourself – it makes her feel worthy of love. And then imagine you post one day having had a nose job. Imagine how that might impact her. We are not alone on this Earth, and though we should always do what is best for us and put our best interests first, we shouldn't forget the impact we might have on our wider community, and the young girls and women who will follow us. If, after everything, you still feel plastic surgery is the only way for you to achieve the happiness and wellbeing you deserve, then please make sure you take the necessary steps to research thoroughly the procedure, the medical centre you plan to have it at and the doctor who will be performing it, their reviews, their experiences with Black patients, the risks, timelines and aftercare. Leave no stone unturned and don't cut corners, especially financially. Ensure you have a support system around you who will be there for you through your recovery and who will embrace the change. Of course, I sincerely hope it works for you!

TAKING IT BLACK

Now let's talk business, baby. The industry of Black beauty cannot be understated. When you bring together make-up, skincare and hair, the exact size of it is hard to calculate but here are just a couple of stats to hammer home the scale of this thing.

Black consumers in the US are estimated to spend over nine times more on beauty and grooming products than their white counterparts. The Black hair care industry has been valued at over 2.5 billion dollars alone (excluding wigs, styling tools and accessories).* Here in the UK, it's estimated by the Black Pound Report that the beauty industry misses out on around 2.7 billion pounds a year by failing to cater for ethnic minority groups. Not only is Black beauty crucial to our culture and our identity, but it's undoubtedly big business.

When you're working with those sorts of numbers in a capitalist society such as ours, it's no surprise at all that everyone wants a piece. And actually, when you dig a little deeper, or if you've spent literally any time shopping around for Black hair products here in the UK for example, it becomes abundantly clear that the resources of Black hair

---

* Hype Hair, https://www.hypehair.com/86642/black-consumers-continue-to-spend-nine-times-more-in-beauty-report/

and beauty are very rarely sold or managed by the Black community. The *McKinsey Quarterly* suggests that Black brands make up only 2.5% of the revenue in the beauty industry, despite Black consumers accounting for more than 11% of the money spent. Never mind how we're represented in the workforces of the non-Black- owned brands that aim to sell us products, too.*

So, with the kind of profit that can be made from us and our custom, it's no surprise that corporations operate on something of a 'don't ask, don't tell' basis when it comes to who's running the show. Big brands have been slowly clocking on to the value of our spending power and nudging themselves into the market, whether that's Pantene, L'Oréal or stockists like Boots and Superdrug finally bringing in diverse product ranges. But without the right perspectives being heard in the boardrooms, these attempts often fall flat, with companies churning out new products for every trend, using language that presents Black beauty as a problem to be fixed and rarely doing the work to investigate the long-term impacts of their chemicals on our health and wellbeing. This is very much a judgement-free zone, but a strong example of this is the conversation that's been happening around chemicals used in relaxers and texturisers for years – ingredients like formaldehyde, mercury, phthalates and others that have been correlated with

---

* McKinsey & Company, https://www.mckinsey.com/industries/consumer-packaged-goods/our-insights/black-representation-in-the-beauty-industry

fibroids in scientific research* and we all know that Black women suffer heavily with fibroids. It's been studied too, as per The Black Women's Health Initiative article, titled 'It's Not Normal: Black Women, Stop Suffering From Fibroids'. Even to this day, despite the questions being raised, there have been very few movements for more strict regulations or policies to stop these harmful products from being sold widely. Without Black people at the helm of these corporations, how do we even begin to demand they prioritise our health and humanity over their profit?

Another ironic aspect of non-Black people wanting and claiming such huge slices of the Black beauty industry is that even while they do it, they often still discriminate against us. If I tried to count on my fingers and toes the number of times I've been followed around a Black hair shop or beauty supply store going back year by year, I'd run out before I reached 2020. And we were even in a pandemic then, so there's really no excuse. It's happened to nearly every Black woman I know. Over in the US, it's the same too. Don't even get me started on the optics of US conglomerates locking up Black beauty products exclusively in their stores – something that only shifted after multiple viral social media callouts and the socio-political reckoning of June 2020. Either way, that was another one of the most memorable and disgusting displays of outright disdain for the very people keeping the lights on in some of these establishments. The experience of merely shopping while

---

* Public Health, https://publichealth.gwu.edu/content/do-harmful-chemicals-consumer-products-fuel-growth-uterine-tumors

Black, in spaces that exist to profit from you, can be deeply unpleasant, overwhelming and even at times triggering. Multiple dark-skinned friends of mine have stories of being offered skin-bleaching products at the till like it was a pack of Extra gum. The micro- and macro-aggressions are never-ending. At the bare minimum, we need more spaces where Black women are empathised with and celebrated before they are accused, judged and demeaned. It's really not too much to ask for.

One of the reasons for this historical dearth in Black-owned hair shops and companies is the simple lack of capital. Both here and in the States, prejudice (backed up by statistics) means that Black founders and business owners are systematically denied more loans and given less money when they get accepted too, as well as finding it harder to raise funds through investment. For example, in the US, Black entrepreneurs are on average lent $35,000 to start businesses versus their white counterparts' $107,000.[*] Starting your own business is also not for the faint-hearted or the small-pocketed. It's a huge privilege and risk to take that can often mean either not making money for a number of years or having to balance an entire other career along-side just to support yourself. That leap is obviously going to be a lot easier to take if you come from a middle-class or financially stable background or are able to access support in the incubation period.

---

[*] McKinsey & Company, https://www.mckinsey.com/industries/retail/our-insights/the-black-unicorn-changing-the-game-for-inclusivity-in-retail

But this is why it's so exhilarating to see an immense new wave of Black-owned businesses launching to take back control of these industries and provide products and experiences grounded in expertise, experience and duty of care. From hair ranges coming from the likes of Ruka hair and influencer Freddie Harrel's brand RadSwan, Black women aren't just claiming their share of the hair industry, they're also innovating in it. They're creating new hair offerings that are practical and protective but that are also unafraid to celebrate and harness the beauty of our natural hair in the process. I remember once going to buy hair for a ponytail and having to clarify to the shop owner multiple times that I wasn't looking for something silky, I was looking for a texture that would mimic my own natural hair pattern. The disbelief and confusion on his face said it all. That and the fact that they didn't have a single curly textured ponytail in the whole shop. These two brands make me so excited for the future of what Black hair culture here in the UK can be – authentic, empowering and accessible.

When it comes to how we nourish our hair and skin – from the likes of the Afro Hair & Skin Co, Bread Beauty Supply, Afrocenchix, Boucleme, Dizziak, Big Hair + Beauty – we are finally being spoiled for choice in the UK. Salons such as Charlotte Mensah's over in west London or Peckham Palms give us places to congregate and pamper ourselves among likeminded energies. Platforms like Carra, Treasure Tress, Curlture and Skin Library provide the space to explore and educate ourselves on our hair and bodies by curating with empathy and thoughtfulness at the heart. The list goes on and on, and I urge you to take that extra second to frequent or virtually visit one of these names the next time you're hovering over your basket on Amazon or picking up supplies at your local chain. From the packaging to the customer service to the genuine effectiveness of the products, I've found making that switch to divest from the places that are more concerned with my money than my wellbeing and instead pour into my own community has improved my relationship to beauty and the products I employ to access it 10 times over.

Black-owned hair shops in London:
  Star Beauty Shop – Islington
  Mr Klass – Tottenham
  Hairitage – Willesden
  Golden Touch – Forest Gate
  TJ Hair & Cosmetics – Walworth
  Peckham Palms – Peckham
  Hairglo – Bromley
  Essence of Nature – Sydenham
  Xsandy's – used to be in Lewisham, now online
  OGB6 Beauty Palace – Crystal Palace
  Bella Hair & Cosmetics – Fulham

I realise we have concentrated on the UK, and at times the US, but it would be foolish of me to not talk about the Black beauty institutions around the globe that are ready to stand up and be counted. In recent years, Black beauty has been empowered by our fellow people and we love to see it. May we never stop. So, without further ado, here they are.

Global Black beauty shops:
  Playhouse Hair – Berlin
  Pat McGrath Labs – Global
  Vernon François – USA
  blackbeautyonline.com/ – online
  Topicals – Global
  Ami Cole – USA
  UOMA Beauty – Global
  IMAN Cosmetics – Global
  Treasure Tress – UK & Europe

'A lot of us aren't told about the fact that a lot of these movements were really centred around Black womanhood and trying to find a safe enough space to celebrate that about ourselves and how different we are, not just in our skin colour but also our sizes and even the way that we think.'
– Enam Asiama

BODY POSITIVITY

Okay, so we've talked about our hair and our skin, plastic surgery and reclaiming ownership over the industry that is Black beauty. Which just leaves the last piece of the puzzle – but it's probably one of the biggest ones. And that is of course the big ol' bag of bones that carries us around *while* we take care of everything else – our bodies.

Black women's bodies have been policed since the dawn of time, it feels like. Whether we're too big in some areas, not big enough in others, showing it off too much or covering it up too much to be deemed desirable, in some spaces our bodies are hypersexualised or seen as objects for other people's gain. In others, they're just plain erased, dismissed and brutalised. These things that are ours that we have for our entire lives, through everything we experience, are used to help support our community, ourselves and our families in a million and one ways on a daily basis, quite literally every step of the way. And while naturally that can mean we take them for granted and forget to acknowledge just how incredible they are, to me personally, I can't really think of any part of me that is more worthy of care, respect and complete unconditional love.

When I say unconditional, I mean *unconditional* – not that I love my body if it performs one specific task well or fits into clothes with tags saying one specific thing or gets me praise from anyone in the outside world. It's the love that says, I love my body because it is my body and as long as that is the case (which is forever) then I will love it regardless. That kind of love can really feel like it's getting harder and harder to achieve in a world that thrives when we set ourselves these requirements and boundaries for our bodies, these targets and goals that it can either succeed or fail to meet in order to be seen as valuable or worth celebrating. Whether that's dropping bags on fashion to make our bodies look a certain way or fitness equipment to tackle certain bits, there's a lot less money to be made from us when we like ourselves just by virtue of the way we already are.

It's no surprise that in the face of all these unrealistic

standards and pressures and burgeoning insecurities, the concept of body positivity has taken on so many different lives and meanings then too, right? For one person, the triumph of it could be as simple as wearing a sleeveless top for the first time in years, even though you feel self-conscious about your arms. For others, it could be posting a pic where you have stretch marks showing instead of editing them out. For someone else, it might look like getting that dessert at dinner and feeling absolutely no type of way about it. As long as these wins are about eradicating the negativity around our physical presence, they are body-positive actions. The name and how the movement has developed can make it seem like if you aren't flaunting your birthday suit in all its glory for the 'gram then you have failed at loving yourself and maybe you aren't as progressive as you think you are. But there really are an infinite number of ways to love yourself.

A movement started by fat Black and Brown women who were historically marginalised, ridiculed and erased for their bodies, the body-positivity movement has definitely been white-washed and diluted for the mainstream in recent years. Instead of using it to platform and centre the people who inspired it in the first place, brands often approach it as a box-ticking exercise, tokenising and alienating plus-size bodies even further as the add-on or afterthought. Others instead try to take the momentum of the movement and use it to cherry-pick from within the community and propel a 'privileged' few forward as the heroes and spokespeople for the movement, which only further erases those that it was created for. For example, only using models of plus sizes who still have an hourglass figure or whose faces are still slim or who are completely bodily able or basically still exist within some of the more rigid beauty proportions of the straight-sized industry in a number of ways. Doing so doesn't give what these companies think it's giving because often these people are the exception to being plus size, not the rule, and platforming them as the worthy ones is just another way to reinforce that there is only one good way to be fat. Which is like only one step less abhorrent than pushing that there is no good way to be fat.

Online spaces however have spawned pockets of true positive representation as people are able to present and showcase their own beauty and others are primed and ready to celebrate it. Model and influencer Enam Asiama remembers when the world of plus-size Instagram first opened up for her and how it compensated for the isolation she was feeling in her day-to-day life: 'On Instagram, I would get all this amazing support and find plus-size people and Black people on there. And it meant I no longer had to care about the [fatphobic] thoughts of the people who were closest to me or that I grew up with ... [Growing up] my friends were always saying things like "if you were to lose this much more weight, you'd be amazing. You're already beautiful but you'd be incredible!" so I was never good enough. But I found this group of people online who were telling me, "girl, you're amazing, we love you, more of your aesthetic, more of your thoughts!" and I just loved it, I felt so comforted.'

I tell you now, once I started to actively investigate who I was following, removing accounts that were making me feel worse about myself (the ones fed to you by the algorithm and catapulted to virality for doing the absolute bare minimum) and replacing them with a beautiful and *vast* range of body types, skin tones, backgrounds, aesthetics, it was just a matter of time before my concept of beauty expanded tenfold. The images that we are faced with every day even subconsciously form such a huge part of our worldview and what we consider to be not just normal but good. These communities can make you feel seen and heard and held in ways that you didn't even know were possible. Like is this really how other people feel all the time? Seeing themselves and the beauty in others who are just like them because everyone in the media is just like them? Mad ting, sad ting.

I think one of the best ways I've found to uplift myself is definitely just by finding the power in uplifting others. For some reason, it feels so much less daunting to start by embracing and empowering something or someone outside of myself, being able to acknowledge their beauty and see it unquestionably. And it's not necessarily a case of projection or making it about you, but it's the practice of surrounding myself with incredible people and images and philosophies and sitting with them in all their glory, before asking myself if I can see how great and wonderful and inspiring all of these people are, what is stopping me from seeing that in myself? Am I not like them? Do I not deserve the same freedoms as them to live authentically and without judgement? What would you say to someone who viewed themself with the harshness that you view yourself?

BODY NEUTRALITY

As a result of the kind of pressure that some can feel to be extremely celebratory or explicitly positive about their body all the time – something that's totally fine but isn't the only way to be – others have leaned towards a new term too, which I love. 'Body neutrality' is very much an offshoot or descendant of the same concept but it's just meant to capture a more pragmatic approach to how we as humans relate to ourselves. It's not uncommon to have a relationship with your body that changes over time; not every day has to feel like bikini day.

Body neutrality is about placing the deserved respect on our bodies as the super crucial and incredible machines that they are, without necessarily focusing so much on their aesthetic value. So instead of saying 'I love my body so much, I love my belly rolls, they are so beautiful', and seeking to reframe the actual standards of beauty to include you, a body neutralist would probably say 'My body is great because it literally carries me around and helps me succeed in life. But I am also more than just my body and how I feel about it may shift from day to day and that is totally okay.' Some people pose it as a step en route to body positivity or a bridge between body negativity and body positivity, but I see it as existing in its own ecosystem. Ultimately, it's just a value structure that wants to remove itself entirely from the economy of aesthetics and beauty that we find ourselves in. It's like saying I love myself because I refuse to let the system that tells me I shouldn't hold any power over me.

I don't just want to 'win' at the game of beauty, right alongside everyone else; I want to take apart the PlayStation.

WELLNESS ACTION POINTS

1. Dedicate one hour per week to self-pamper time. That could be a 10-minute face massage every night before bed, 5 minutes of morning affirmations in the mirror, taking 30 minutes on a Sunday to re-moisturise your ends or booking in that nail, brows or lashes appointment.

2. List five things that you love about yourself right now and wouldn't change for the world. Make an effort to find ways to celebrate and pay homage to those parts of yourself today. If it's your hands, get a cute manicure. If it's your legs, buy yourself a fancy, good-smelling moisturiser and take your time lotioning them. If it's your laugh, watch some stand-up comedy or put your favourite sitcom on. If it's your smile, pop that Fenty Beauty lip gloss on and get to grinning. Sit in that feeling of warmth and luxury.

3. Cleanse your timeline. Have a scroll and browse through your social media and unfollow or mute any account that you feel ignites negative feelings inside you about your body and the way you look. Do some research and follow three people who promote body positivity and body neutrality in a truly representative and authentic way.

Eight

BLACK MOTHERHOOD

Okay, I know what some of you are thinking: 'I'm not a mother; this one doesn't apply to me. Next.' But please don't skip this chapter! I promise you that I'm writing this as much for you as I am the next reader who *does* already have children and identifies with the title. You just have to trust me.

Unfortunately, I feel like society doesn't do enough to teach young women and girls about the actual realities of motherhood. We have these romanticised portrayals of it and this language that reduces it to 'having kids' or 'having babies' rather than the full force and responsibility of raising humans. I think while many of our preconceptions and concerns revolve around pregnancy as this strange time for our bodies, we often romanticise the idea of becoming a mum as this opportunity to relive our own childhoods or play dress up. Obviously, a lot of us understand it beyond these cutesy aspects, but still, I feel like the vast majority of motherhood's complexities go unspoken.

And ultimately where society fails to keep us up to speed, life takes the chance to give us a rude awakening. Becoming a mother is one of the most incredible things a person can do, never mind that in many contexts it's also considered a privilege. But it is also a lifechanging event, from how it transforms our reality to how it quite literally transforms our bodies and our minds too. And speaking from experience, it's unlike anything I could have fathomed before it happened directly to me. But even if it's impossible to grasp in theory, I really do think there's so much strength in trying to. In opening the lines of truthful communication between those who have undergone these experiences and those who are willing to listen to us.

As I ruminate on the emotional and physical rollercoaster that has been my own personal motherhood journey so far, one thing that surfaces is that I felt like I definitely lost myself. From things as simple as picking out an outfit to remembering the most basic piece of information; not gonna lie, I've breathed new life to the saying, 'you'd lose your own head if it wasn't attached to your body', and even worse, I've genuinely worried about the risk of pulling a David Cameron in a cloud of forgetfulness and leaving my son somewhere! No matter how much you think you've heard about the elusive concept of 'baby brain', you have no idea, sis. A woman at an event once whispered to me while I was still pregnant that baby brain was real, before adding that it doesn't actually ever leave. And while that probably wasn't what I wanted to hear at that moment in time, she was absolutely right.

Every day on this path is one of healing and recovery, and week on week I feel myself getting stronger and stronger, and if not stronger, then at least more comfortable and confident in my new forever role. I'll never return to the

Chloé that I was pre-October 2020. Instead, I'm making my way to a Chloé 2.0, who is much stronger than the woman I was before. She's self-aware and she has a wealth of new responsibilities. She can't just get up and roll on with her morning; she has a little human who relies on her, knows her, wants her and needs her. No woman will ever understand the meaning of clingy until she has a child. It's real. And the gravity of that is cemented with each passing day and the purity of the look in his eyes staring right back into mine. In those moments, everything that has come before becomes secondary and he is my only priority. The routines and the knowledge that predate your little miracle disintegrate into the background and your past self becomes nearly unrecognisable. I've learnt that it's okay to miss that, and better still, that it's okay to be open about it. So, ultimately, while I lost a version of myself, I found another through that metamorphosis.

Another key thing to remember about becoming a mother is that *everyone's experiences are different*. Yes, as women, trans men and non-binary people, we can have a shared understanding of what comes with the title 'mother' – the long nights, the sore nipples, the joy of holding your child or the vulnerability of parenting and not knowing what to do in the moment – we will also all have completely different journeys, from getting pregnant to being pregnant and then to raising your children. It's like each of us are headed to the same place, but none of us are taking the same form of transport or the same route. This is so important to remind yourself, because it can often feel like you aren't doing mothering 'right' or the 'best' it can be done, but that's simply not true. Of course, it's great to share tips, tricks and knowledge, but you absolutely don't have to take it all on board. Just as in any part of life or wellness, you have to find the methods that work for you and that allow you to feel joy, happiness and peace.

Then there's this idea of the 'bounce back', a phrase used to describe the physical and lifestyle rebound you're supposed to undergo to return to your pre-pregnancy body and weight and lifestyle as if nothing ever happened. When in fact, everything has happened and changed, and you literally created a life within your own body in under a year and, to be honest, we still don't spend nearly enough time freaking out about how ridiculous that even is!!! But whether you believe in the idea or not, you are bound to be peppered with roughly a thousand variations of the same question: when do you plan to return to work? What about your career? Have you got the hang of 'it'? (Whatever *it* is.) What next? How many more? How soon until . . .? The list goes on and on.

And between figuring out how to stay present in an ever-changing social landscape, maintaining the life and spark in your own relationships and figuring out this entirely new set of rules and roles you are playing without a definitive handbook, the word I'd use to describe it all is just . . . stretched. Once again, we have to prepare and remind ourselves that there is no such thing as a linear or even cyclical journey when it comes to motherhood. In this case, that means there really is no going back, only forging forward. And as Black mothers, that trusty old phrase of 'working twice as hard' isn't limited to the traditional workspace. And though money and time can help ease the path, we all have to arm ourselves with the expectations and tools at every point of this journey to feel aware and at peace with what's to come. Truly, I've realised this is the only method of survival . . . and that's to adapt. And even for those of us who don't consider themselves to be mothers or maybe don't ever plan to be in the future, there are so many aspects of Black motherhood that can help us on our own journey to advocate best for ourselves and for others around us.

MOTHERING WHILE BLACK

Though our contexts, ideas and even basic understanding of what falls under the umbrella are often extremely different, it's very hard to argue with the fact that modern-day parenting and motherhood, especially where it intersects with race, is very intentional. When you consider the aspects of choice, of heritage, of family structures and of gender, Black motherhood in particular can be seen as a huge celebration and foundation of our community. It's the story of so many of us, both living and those who have passed.

And you could even argue that to be a Black mother is a political statement in and of itself. For me personally, it says, 'I am' and 'I have made my choice' loud and clear for the world to see and do with it what they will. And sadly, we don't have to look very far back in history at all to begin to witness the concepts of consent and choice unravelling before our very eyes as they pertain to Black motherhood.

And it's all the more reason to emphasise that in spite of that, here we are, here *I am*, standing in and honouring the lineage of Black mothers.

In the book *Birthing Black Mothers*, Black feminist theorist Jennifer C. Nash examines how the figure of the 'Black mother' has become a powerful political category, and I believe the Black mother experience begins way before one Black mother has her first child. In my humble opinion, this moment, realisation, awakening even, begins for the female when she is very young and first aware that her gender is female. In this moment, she will quickly learn what the world expects of her and what her duty is within the household she is raised in (note: hardship). I, for one, also believe that this is where female empowerment as a tradition (whether positive, negative or neutral) is handed down from generation to generation, or where it should begin. A lot of our understanding of motherhood is learnt from how we are each mothered (or not). Whether our own mother is cold, distant, warm, loving, strict, understanding, absent, present, it all adds to our understanding of what being a mum means. And while your own mum is a complex human being with influences, both good and bad, all around her, this can sometimes not give a clear view of what mothering should and shouldn't look like. How we are mothered or parented can have a huge impact on us, which is why therapy can be incredibly helpful as a way to unpack our understanding of parenting before we raise a child of our own and make similar mistakes.

Of course, we can and will go into generational and childhood trauma because as you well know, there is little room to escape this when discussing Black history and Black parenting. But I would like to add very early on in the conversation, that in this same way, and as a Black mother myself, while we often parent as a priority due to said need for survival, legacy and even as an act of resistance, it leaves little room for the sustenance we need to be consistent and also to simply breathe for ourselves, rather than just ensuring our offspring and families breathe (and breathe well). And this is where we need to show up for ourselves and bring the conversation back to wellness, or if you like *mother's wellness*.

Often, especially in the West, you'll see Black mothering placed in direct comparison to white motherhood and parenting, a natural human practice but a vast oversimplification. Ultimately, comparison is only fair where the playing fields are, too. Survival, resistance and hardship are by no means the only or defining features of the Black

'My mama was my first reminder of strength and guidance and how to be unapologetic about the way she meditates and prays and taps into those areas of herself . . . My mum is a prayer warrior, she really taps into what she needs and what her family needs and what her loved ones need. Even if she's met a stranger on the street, she'll pray for them and think about them and try to nurture them.' – Enam Asiama

experience, but the context of extending and expanding our lifelines and our families within and against these often destructive structures and confines is a context that cannot be tossed aside. And our power is in defiantly loving and connecting and growing in spite of it all.

Like our non-Black counterparts, we want the very best for our children despite being told in many different ways that this simply isn't possible or deserved. Maybe it's all the subliminal and increasingly public hurdles and obstacles that we face every day and attribute to us the 'superwoman' status that none of us asked for. But does anyone really know what we go through? How to exist and hopefully thrive as a Black mother? What does it look like to be struggling with the pressures of raising children as a Black person? How do we not lose it? And if we do lose it, how do we find our way back?

And don't get me started on labels. None of these apparent badges of freedom and choice – e.g. 'working mum', 'stay-at-home mum', 'homemaker', 'housewife', 'single mum' – seem to accurately describe the actual value of mothering, particularly as a Black mother.

To be a warrior for your children, the backbone, the provider, the nurturer, the friend, the safety, the teacher that prepares them for the world but also the respite and the sanctuary for them, too. In short, being a Black mother really doesn't come with any medals or credit and even representation in big big 2023, but it is an achievement. So, if you are a mother – and in particular a *Black* mother – reading this, possibly struggling in one way or not, please reward yourself in the knowledge that you are mighty and you are seen and validated through all of the pages of this book and beyond. The community appreciates you. For those of you not yet on this journey, feel powerful in the knowledge you are doing something incredible and vital. Mothering comes in many forms, and you are just as much a part of this puzzle as anyone else. There is so much good that comes with being a mother, and that includes considering the position and we should take courage and strength in that.

In contrast to the usual image of Black mothers in the media as either struggling and not up to par or as these tragic heroes, Nash unpacks how many of our most visible figures – the likes of Beyoncé, Serena Williams, Michelle Obama, to name a few – actually represent themselves. Not as cautionary tales but as blueprints: empowered, complexly textured, hard and soft, powerful and vulnerable energy sources. Being a Black mother is about so much more than loving and nurturing your child, which of course is the priority. We also have to equip our children with the tools to navigate a world that will quickly judge them for what they look like over their talent, character or experience while also propping ourselves and others simultaneously. It is the precarious balancing act of our reality and our wildest dreams.

I think the concept of the Superwoman Syndrome is a particularly pressing complex for Black mothers who are told by the world that struggle is

> 'My mum has always said to me and my sister that she wants to learn from us as much as we can learn from her.'
> – Char Ellesse

part of the journey and that we should be our own last priority. Coined by Marjorie Hansen Shaevitz in 1984 in her book of the same name, it's a term used to describe a woman who deprioritises her own needs with the goal of reaching perfection in each role she inhabits, often completely unrealistically. Not because she isn't capable, but because the standards she sets for herself are impossibly high and she will very rarely consider her wellness as a vital part of attaining her goal.

While I'm all for pushing and breaking boundaries, exploring multiple passions and wanting the best for ourselves, I'm here to remind you that motherhood is not the place to exercise your biggest superhero fantasies. The 'pouring from an empty cup' saying exists for a reason, and even if you can't see it, when you deplete your reserves in the frantic pursuit of all-round perfectionism, it's not just you but also your child that feels the consequences of that. To be the best mothers that we can be, we have to accept and love ourselves as we are presently, as wholly as we can and strive to love our children – wholeheartedly and unconditionally. There is no world in which we can and will do it all, and our perfectionism can actually get in the way of us doing what's best and being our most human.

And as time passes, it will never stop shifting, becoming more and more of a conversation as we learn from generations raised in different worlds to us with subsequently different perspectives. The beauty of generations flowing forward through history is hopefully a constant progression of our lives and opportunities as the years go on and on. We go through what we go through and overcome to ensure that we don't have to again and neither do our children. And what's so special about that is that eventually it means there will be a bunch of things for us to learn from our children too. And that's not a symbol of failure but instead one of overwhelming success.

WELLNESS ACTION POINTS

As a (fairly) new Black mother myself, my final word must be that without any shadow of doubt, I am devoted to seeing our Black children soar – as the incredible artist Lina Iris Viktor highlighted in her 2022 Hayward Gallery exhibition: 'there are Black people in the future!' – and in that same breath, for our children to soar, we must too. Our very existence has proved the great jobs our mothers collectively did previously but in order to move forward in this exact greatness, we need to slightly pivot our output to include ourselves in the vision of success, so our children can follow suit and do the same.

Write down your answers to these questions and keep your responses to document how your own relationship with motherhood shifts over the years:

1. What's one thing you wish you could thank your mother for?
2. What's something you wish she knew?
3. What does wellness in Black motherhood mean to you? How do you actively practise this yourself? What can you do better?

4. What are the things you love and value about yourself *outside* of being a mother? What do you not want to lose once you become/while being a mother?

5. What do you want your children to know, acknowledge, remember and pass on once you are gone?

Nine

CREATING A COMMUNITY

> 'Sometimes, working to the brink feels like the
> only option. And for many Black people, it is.
> That's where community comes in – or at least,
> it should.'
>
> – Kathleen Newman-Bremang

Often, when we think of wellness, we see it as a solo mission – a path we have to face entirely on our own in order for it to be 'real'. There's this idea that if your happiness or wellbeing is reliant on someone else then it can't be legitimate. And in many ways, there is truth in that. If your wellbeing relies on someone else outside of yourself, it becomes conditional rather than self-sufficient, meaning that its success or lifespan can end up depending on things outside of your control. Think of a codependent relationship where, yeah, when you're together everything feels right and good in the world, but the moment you separate or things between you start to lose your shine, it's hard for you to cope without that other person. In times like those, it's vital to have the tools to not just self-soothe but to build yourself back up again. In that sense, there's always an argument for making sure that you are able to thrive on your own and determine your wellbeing for yourself. To do the things you want to do and be the person you want to be without anyone else's permission.

But at the same time, we don't exist in a vacuum. Even with all the independence and inner strength in the world, at our core we as humans are inherently social animals! And to ignore that would be a huge disservice to that basic instinct of ours to want to form connections with others and live in a community. Pretty much since the dawn of time, humans have existed in groups and tapped into individual strengths to construct well-oiled societal machines – hunters, gatherers, nurturers, fighters. Community has served as a means to allow us to not feel like we have all of the answers ourselves; where we lack someone else might shine. And when balanced carefully alongside an innate sense of self and independence separate from these groups we participate in, community can be a key player in a life of wellness too.

To me, community is as much about giving as it is about receiving – it's what is borne out of the difference between reliance and reciprocity. To be a good community member, you have to ask yourself not just what you are getting out of the spaces you occupy but also what you can contribute. And that's not just because it makes it fairer or feels like the

> 'Service to others is the rent you pay for your room here on Earth.'
> – Shirley Chisholm

right thing to do but because being an active participant, with a role to play in these micro-societies, is one of the keys to feeling more valued and present in the world around you.

BUILDING COMMUNITY

Building community can be a truly terrifying prospect, let's be honest. Admitting that you need things from other people that you can't get from yourself – be that comfort, support, friendship – is a step towards vulnerability that can feel really hard to take. Especially if it's something you haven't necessarily experienced before, or worse, have had a negative experience with already. Sometimes it can feel like everyone in the world has found their tribe except you and no matter how hard you try to fit into certain spaces, none feel like a natural fit.

I think we can often have these ideas of what a community can and should look like. At a macro level, they're these big, sprawling crowds of people who all get along and stand firmly on this common ground that unites them. On a more micro level, it's a friendship group where everyone looks like they belong together, they speak the same cultural language, have the same interests and tastes; they just 'get' it – shit, their outfits might even be coordinated. But in reality, community comes in so many more unexpected shapes and sizes. It's the group chat or DM created by you with 10 other people in your field of work to brain dump all the questions you think sound too stupid for the main feed. It's that Facebook group that you muted the notifications for on your street because Aileen at number three won't stop complaining about someone putting their recycling in her bin. It's the familiar faces you see on the cramped bus every morning to work and exchange knowing glances with when the couple next to you have their third fight of the week. It's the guy at the coffee shop who gives you your tea for free because it's your fifth time coming in this week, and he knows your bank account must be yelling. Sometimes the greatest community you find doesn't always look like you'd expect it to.

When we find these miniscule bursts of connection with others that are often completely untethered, these are the sorts of things I think we hold on to, nurture and build into the most natural and organic kinds of community for ourselves – the ones that sprout with no provocation or expectation. Find the people that you gravitate towards naturally and take the first step to put yourself out there with them. Go on a friend date and start to build a connection. Ask that stranger what their name is or how their day has been. Community doesn't need to start like bootcamp at The X Factor back in the day where they'd select random unsuspecting teens and lump them together and force them to pick a name. It can be as simple as two people reaching out in a storm of flakiness and strangers getting to know each other.

Community is happening around you all of the time, it's how society continues to function. But it's down to us to make those interactions as rich and human as they possibly can be.

Creating A Community

As Black women, we spend a lot of time occupying spaces that weren't necessarily shaped with us in mind – whether it's at school, in the workplace or just existing out in the world. And though we come from so many different walks of life and have lived vastly different realities, we have these threads that often run through our stories and connect us to one another. There's a really beautiful mutual understanding and visibility that comes from our kinship.

I think one of the biggest catalysts for community is the act of sharing. For many of us who feel tied to these notions of strength and independence, vulnerability is the most daunting concept. We don't want to be a bother or a burden to anyone, and when we are, we sometimes struggle to believe that the people we rest our worries at the feet of are actually going to be able to pull through for us. We can be so used to figuring things out on our own and being let down that it starts to make us isolated from the communities that are already around us and eager to be the support system we need. But at my roughest points, I've learnt that it's only in trusting others and allowing them to see our full selves that

> 'Black womanhood has taught me that we are truly connected. We share the same experiences, we have the same traumas, and when you have something like that it makes you closer and gives you that sense of community. It's also learning the ways in which we navigate through those things.'
>
> – Enam Asiama

we can really bond on a deeper and more enriching level and start to nurture the connections that we all crave deep down. Finding people that you can do that with safely who can make you feel held and seen in at least some of the nuances of your identity is so precious. For me, that process started with just reaching out and asking for help on the smallest things to start with, asking a friend to come shopping with me or for their opinion on a work situation – just finding ways to let them into my inner world bit by bit. In return, they would start to do the same more and more and it became this spider's web of women who were able to prop each other up and help guide each other through life together. The lesson I learnt here is that not only does taking the leap to share benefit you but it also benefits the people around you. Regardless of what that little voice in your brain is telling you, the people around you love you and care about you, and not only do they want to see you thrive, but they'd be honoured to play even a small role in that journey right alongside you.

Another great way to build community is through your own hobbies and interests. In this capitalist world, we don't always have the luxury of time to spend alone, with others or just even generally on the things that we love. But what I will say is that when we do find those windows of opportunity, why not find a way to combine all three. One of the few upsides or symptoms of the pandemic was that it eliminated a lot of the extra time-consumers we were living with, for example, commuting or leaving the house generally. And in that time, it was fascinating to see the different things we discovered to fill those gaps in our lives with new hobbies and activities. Some got hardcore into puzzles; others were sourdough connoisseurs. I think there were probably a lot of badly knitted jumpers gifted for Christmas that year too. But ultimately, I think some of that whimsy and playfulness around doing things purely for the love of doing them enriches our lives in ways that you only usually get to have as a child. Think about the things that you would fill your days with on the off chance you won the lottery and had all the free time in the world, and find ways to fit those joys into your routine now somehow. Because this life is really too short to keep putting off the activities that fulfil us in the hopes of some theoretical future that isn't coming. The only moment we are promised is the one we're in right now, so we may as well do something good with it. And the best thing about these hobbies is that they often come pre-attached with communities of their own. Whether it's a local crochet club, a pottery studio or joining a pole-dancing class, pursuing these hobbies is a really great way to end up in spaces with people who share the same loves as you. It's an automatic connector. And it doesn't even have to cost you money; you could look to build your own online community where you're able to share resources and ask advice from others or just meet up to experiment and learn new skills together.

The last thing I'll say about the idea of finding a tribe is definitely an overused phrase, but why fix it if it ain't broke? That phrase is *quality over quantity*. When you look on socials (or even just watch a lot of TV), it can be really easy to end up thinking to yourself . . . does everyone have more friends than me? You'll see folks out at bottomless brunches CONSTANTLY, attending weddings every weekend and jumping around to multiple motives in one night, and it can start to feed into your very natural and normal feelings of FOMO (fear of missing out) or general social insecurity. But I'm here to tell you that first of all, just because you have a thought doesn't make it automatically true – at some point in their lives, I promise you, nearly *everyone* has felt that way. It's an optical illusion. Of course, when social media is literally a slideshow of every other person's social calendar and highlights and you consume that content on a daily – or hourly – basis while living your normal, unfiltered, fully comprehensive life of things like laundry and chores and emails, the accumulated impact of that is going to feel like you're the only one losing out. Like everyone is thriving while you're heating up your microwave meal. But when you put it into perspective you have to realise that we just aren't seeing the non-shiny bits of everyone else's existence and you are not doomed to unpopularity just because your social calendar is not b2b2b2b with house parties and dates.

The second and more important aspect of this is that it also really does not matter what anybody else is up to at all. Let me repeat that, it *really* does not matter what anybody else is getting up to. So long as you feel held and supported and are nurturing your own relationships, whether there are four, five, six or twenty of them, your community is just as valid and precious as the next one. Having more 'friends' does not inherently equal more happiness or more fun or even more support. In fact, sometimes it defo means the opposite, if we're being real. More often than not, the communities centred around appearances and visibility are some of the most surface-level and unfulfilling, especially if they aren't connections made for genuine purposes or with genuine compatibility. Don't be fooled! Focusing on the quality and depth of your own connections with others without watching what other people are doing is a fast-track key to success, I swear. Do the things you want to do, with the people that you want to do them with. Find the best friendship fits for you and your own path in life, water them well and they'll have the ability to grow into exactly what you need. These things take time. And if after a while you actively feel the gaps in your community, take the necessary steps to reach out to others and fill them.

DIGITAL COMMUNITIES

One of my favourite aspects of community is its ability to transcend the physical. In the age of social media where so much can go very left in the digital sphere, there are seemingly limitless connections to be made with like-minded people. If you're feeling isolated or unseen by the people you come across on a daily basis, or you live somewhere where not that many people can relate to your experience, places like Instagram and Twitter can become a real saving grace. The ways that we are able to express creativity, humour and even our pain through these languages are limitless, using these digital spheres as a place to laugh together, grieve together, sometimes to be toxic as hell (let's be honest) but also to organise, effect change and demand better from the world.

One of the biggest, of course, if we can even still call it one community rather than hundreds of micro-communities, is definitely Black Twitter. It's the glorious manifestation of pockets of Black folks across the entire diaspora that consistently locate and generate so much joy and humour for so many of us and have a cultural impact even further beyond their immediate reach. From acronyms like 'TFW' to phrases like 'lit' and 'fleek' back in the day, so much of the new language of younger generations started off right there on Black Twitter, with AAVE and a lot of queer communities to thank, too. When you think about the phrases popping off now even, so many originated from drag queen culture too: for example, 'serving . . .', 'it's giving . . .', 'slay' and without these beautiful blurred boundaries between all of our intersecting identities, who knows if these subcultures could have had such a huge effect on the mainstream.

Another great side effect of online communities is being able to curate your digital experience to feel as safe and inclusive as possible. Even in terms of the kinds of images we consume on a daily basis, platforms and collectives that seek to disrupt the mainstream help us form more healthy images of ourselves and unlearn the toxic standards. You might not know even five or ten people in your everyday life who have the same lived experience as you yet, but through platforms like Instagram, you can dive deep into rabbit holes and either connect with others looking for the same, or at least expose yourself to content and inspiration far beyond your immediate vicinity that helps you see the beauty in your own community and shows you you're not alone. I still remember the day I realised I actually didn't need to follow hundreds of accounts of women who had bodies and skin and hair that I could never achieve and ultimately wasn't that interested in pining after anymore. What pops up on my feed is well within my control and when I started to search for images that felt more true and authentic to me, my tastes and what I wanted to be in life (namely unapologetic, genuine, well-rounded and holistic), it played such a role in positively reinforcing that unlearning process for me and normalising new ideas of beauty and strength outside of what the mainstream media was still funnelling.

BEWARE: COMMUNITIES THAT DON'T SERVE YOU

Like we were talking about earlier, there can be a really thin line between finding community with people that complement you in life and entering into the territory of codependency, both in relationships and in friendships. It's crucial not to allow your desire to belong somewhere lead you to accepting anything. Take it from me, being stuck within communities that don't serve you can be a huge drain on your energy and time and stunt your own personal growth too. The societal pressure and shame surrounding being alone plays a massive part in this.

Here are some things I keep in mind when temperature-checking the communities I partake in:

Does this community encourage you to share your perspective or try to shape it?
Some of the most distinct and recognisable communities

can often come with these identity requirements attached that they look to impress upon the members who take part. Outside of the basic moral ones like equal rights for all, intersectional feminism and more universal social justice beliefs, I urge you to check in with yourself about whether the community you're a part of feels like they're embracing the real you as you are or if they are applying pressure in big or small ways to change and shape you. Do you feel like you have to dress or look a certain way? Do you put your ideas or opinions down? Do you feel free to share them in the first place? Often these communities with more obvious markers of 'belonging' can feel like the most desirable or exclusive clubs that you want to be a part of, but ultimately your communities are supposed to be able to meet you where you're at and empower you to live your best life, not make you feel inadequate or silenced.

How do they talk about and care for people in their absence? A big telltale sign of how someone treats you or speaks about you when you're not in the room is looking at how they do so with others around you. As a general rule of thumb, if people in the group gossip or make jokes at the expense of those who aren't there to defend themselves, chances are it doesn't only happen when you're there to see it. It's probably behaviour that they exhibit whenever you're around, and besides the fact that it's just generally bad vibes, you can also assume that they probably do the same thing when you're not there too.

How do I feel in the aftermath?

There's no better way to get a grasp of someone's effect on you than by taking stock of your energy levels and general demeanour directly after spending time with them. Not every social interaction you have is going to go perfectly and there are of course a ton of external factors that contribute to this too, but looking out for patterns of behaviour and emotions can definitely be a first step to acknowledging a toxic situation. Also, if you find yourself leaning towards introversion versus extroversion, that's important to take into account too as you may just find hanging out with all people quite tiring! Only you can truly gauge how you feel. But after spending time with this group of people do you feel energised, lighter with a more positive outlook on life and the world, or are you a little more tired, deflated, in need of a rest or downtime to recover? Often when we're around people that we aren't totally compatible with, we can end up overexerting ourselves and almost performing for them. In the moment it can feel fine and maybe even fun, but afterwards and in the long run, those types of connections can feel really exhausting or superficial. And I have to emphasise, incompatibility is definitely not a reason to cut people off on its own, but it's something to be aware of when thinking about the kinds of friendships you have and the expectations or boundaries you can place on them. Which leads pretty neatly on to my next point.

R.E.S.P.E.C.T.

Can I rely on them? As I just discussed, not all friendships are created equally and not every friend is going to be that call in the middle of the night, by your side, ride or die. Does that mean they deserve to be blacklisted? Absolutely not. But regardless of that, this question is more about evaluating the respect and care with which those you're in community with treat the bonds you have, even if you're only at that brunch once every six months level of friendship. When they say they'll do something for you, do they do it? If you ask them to respect your wishes on something private or sensitive, are those boundaries kept intact or are they disregarded? Do you feel safe to express how you feel about a problematic situation if and when it occurs? Even when it comes to exchanges that can feel small or inconsequential – the things that you tell yourself not to overreact about – there's such a thing as 'death by a thousand cuts'. Loosely translated from the ancient Chinese torture tactic of 'lingchi', it's evolved into the idea that a whole barrage of small but painful encounters or events can equal a lingering death or avalanche into this larger negative impact. Don't invalidate the pain or betrayals that you feel just because you don't think they'd be considered significant enough by some societal standard.

WELLNESS ACTION POINTS

1. Reach out to a friend you haven't seen in a while and schedule a catch-up coffee. With the beauty of this modern world, this could even be virtual or a phone call; it doesn't have to be something that's scheduled nine weeks down the line when you both next have a free morning. Ask them how 'they are and listen to the answer. Follow up with

more questions and don't be afraid to share what you're going through too – don't brush it off and assume they don't want to hear about it.

2. Find one activity that you can do on a weekly basis that requires involvement from someone else other than you. Living in overpopulated cities that force us to balance busy lifestyles with so many demands on our time and resources means that we often get really used to our independence and pride ourselves on the ability to handle it all. And don't get me wrong, taking charge of your own life and being able to thrive in your own bubble is a really admirable strength to have! But if you've noticed that you've fallen into a pattern of not needing anyone other than yourself for your week to go as planned, maybe look for ways you can fold more community-based activities into your routine and ease yourself back into those kinds of dynamics. It could be a personal training session where you need someone to spot you on your reps, a pottery class where you're being taught or something as simple as offering to complete a task or errand for someone else or asking them to do the same for you. It's those little interactions that can really help ground us in and remind us of the space we have within even our smallest communities (our families or friendship circles), that you are needed by others, and you have needs that you can ask to be met. The heavy load of this life is one that's meant to be shared and there's no shame in that.

3. List three key strengths of your own and ways that
   you can harness them to better a community that
   you're a part of. Sometimes it can feel like we don't
   know where to start when it comes to changing
   or contributing to the world around us. You see
   someone else doing something cool and think 'if
   only I could do that', or maybe someone posts an
   event and you wish you could go but actually don't
   really have a reason why you can't ... Take this
   as a little prompt to help you home in on potential
   ways for you to build or find a community near
   you. If you had to rank your top three stand-out
   qualities, what would they be? Are you really
   funny, sociable, strategic, a great planner, articulate or have great visual style? If you're struggling,
   start by looking at the things you enjoy most and
   then the reasons why you do. Once you have those
   three qualities, write them down spaced out on a
   page and start to branch off ways that you might
   be able to utilise those within your own communities. For example, if you're a master organiser,
   why don't you plan a fun day out for a group of
   your friends that you haven't seen for a while. If
   you're really sociable, consider volunteering at your
   local charity shop every once in a while. If you're a
   strategic thinker, think about mentoring someone!
   There are so many ways to form small moments of
   community and bridge these gaps between people
   today that sometimes feel far too big to conquer.

Ten

SELF-ADVOCACY

Self-advocacy as a term alone feels pretty daunting. As soon as you hear it, it gives off the vibe of something complicated, serious and maybe even a little painful. But realistically, it's a concept we come into contact with again and again throughout our lives: from when you go to see your GP with a health concern and they tell you 'no, you can't have that referral – once again, all you need for your recurring symptoms are some painkillers and bed rest' or when you go to a restaurant and they bring out a meal you didn't order. (I firmly believe there are only two kinds of people in this world – those who will send that meal back with absolute swiftness and all the confidence in the world, and those who will just pretend everything's fine and eat it anyway, maybe even convincing themselves that it was a better choice than the meal they actually ordered in the first place.) But in those situations where you might feel unheard or not cared for, being able to advocate for yourself in a way that's clear and effective while also skirting the line of what's reasonable and compassionate towards others can be a really tricky balance to master. Especially as we are people navigating through systems that often don't account for us, and in some cases are literally set up for us to fail or paint us as difficult for demanding the bare minimum. In fact, the worst part is that the very systems that tell us we shouldn't ask for more or convince us that we're not deserving of it, are usually the systems that need to be listening to us a whole lot harder, making it all the more difficult to pull them up on their failures.

I, too, was once that person who had a lot of 'mouth' but then when I found myself in what I perceived as adult or serious environments like the local council authority, my GP or the hospital, especially when I was pregnant, not only did I not know the correct way to self-advocate or use my voice, I wasn't expected to. I remember once, a while before starting thy.self, I found myself in a dead-end job. I felt personally attacked by my employers and directors on a constant basis, and to cut a long story short, I was on the brink of self-devastation, depression and worse. Luckily, I had a partner who was ready to support me and clearly show me how to self-advocate in a way that as a Black man surrounded by white family his whole life, it came as second nature. After watching me come home deflated after failing to convince a revolving doctor in my local GP practice that I needed more support, I needed a sick note, I needed time away from that environment and I needed it now, he marched me straight back there the next day, sat holding my hand the entire time and directed the next GP to do exactly what I felt I needed. He wasn't aggressive; he was assured, and not once did he move out of his seat or raise his voice. I still have to stop in awe of that moment. On the outside, he was never even that guy. I had never seen anything like it; he was poised, yo! And to make it better (or worse), I had never felt backed in that way before. Like my whole life, I had never felt advocated for in that way. The way I felt after that was unreal, secure, loved and optimistic about my future. Thankfully, that energy rubbed off on me once I got my shit together (only to be knocked again a few years later, but you know life). With that awareness, sis, let me tell you, I contest bills I know the man shouldn't be sending in my name and I can reciprocate love from my community while demanding fairer pay, wellness and visibility.

I think my most recent memory of self-advocacy was when I had to advocate for myself and my unborn child against the UK's failing NHS. When I was five-months pregnant and suffering extreme trauma, I received a call – a routine call, mind you – from a registrar at my chosen London hospital, who randomly asserted that I couldn't and wouldn't be allowed to have a water birth. Not because I have a risky background – it was my first baby, I have no prior health issues and the hospital provided this service free of charge – but wait for it . . . because she deemed me 'obese' after glancing at my notes. Me. ME! Of all people, obese! And to top it off, she wasn't even someone certified to be in the delivery room, let alone tell me what kind of birth I could or could not have or anything about my body. One thing about me is, you can't play with me or my child. Period. After taking her details, and her being blissfully unaware of what was coming next, I called my midwife and left a very urgent message. By the next week I was meeting the head of the antenatal department, and post-water birth (during which I caught my own baby with my bare hands), another five months later, I was invited back to sit on a board deciding the department's next safeguarding team members. If that isn't self-advocating as a Black woman in an institutionally racist country – yes, I said it – and taking ownership of my body, my experiences and my child's wellbeing in his crucial first hours of entering the world, I don't know what is. I don't need a medal; I just need you to swallow up and bathe in this energy and show up the same for yourself and other people you know. I still don't have my PhD, and I don't always know how to code-switch when my temper is brewing, but I can contest anything I think is unfair and negotiate the best deal for myself. And so can you!

Now, it doesn't make sense to talk about advocating for yourself and your career without addressing the massive elephant in the room, one that goes by the name of Imposter Syndrome. It's a term that we're hearing more and more these days, but I still think it's important to really unpack what it is and what it means for our day-to-day life, how it might impact the way we move through the world and how exactly we can begin to overcome it.

And as if that isn't hard enough, that feeling of unworthiness doesn't just stay as an internal monologue. There are so many different ways that Imposter Syndrome can begin to manifest itself in our lives too beyond just the voice in your own head. Whether that's a distrust of others and their praise of you, their ability to believe in you and even their willingness to help you, it can make you retreat even further into yourself for fear of being found out as someone who isn't qualified or worthy. In the long term, those doubts can start to colour your every interaction, making you hard to reach emotionally because you refuse to take compliments or listen to others' more positive perceptions of you, even when meant with the best of intentions. In other areas, it can lead to burnout due to the setting of totally unreasonable goals and expectations in order to 'prove yourself' or impress others, the endless search for perfection in your work and a constant need to overprepare and become an expert in every aspect of life you tackle (though – spoiler alert! – even when you are an expert, you still won't feel like one). It's a very specific and lonely battle that eventually threatens to bring your relationships and your external presence down into the riptide too if you let it.

Speak to most women, and on a good day, they will openly admit to feeling this way at some point or another, if not frequently. Your girl crush or favourite online career baddie . . . yup, her too. Negative, all-encompassing mindsets tend to encroach when they are not wanted and particularly affect Black women for a number of known and unknown reasons. An unknown source once told me that sometimes Imposter Syndrome has a way of affecting the most outwardly successful people in society the most. That may be because they feel as if they might have the most to lose, but it's more than likely because even with a perceived amount of unchallenged success, a mind, whoever it belongs to, has a negative bias, a familial tendency to focus on and be largely impacted by negative experiences. In short, it's human nature.

Imposter Syndrome is arguably one of the biggest phenomenons and dangers of our generation. We are so comfortable calling it out, and in truth, it's one of the most demanded (yet uncomfortable) workshops I deliver for thy.self, but I have always questioned why so many women are affected by Imposter Syndrome. And breaking down the female demographic further, how does this specifically affect Black women, and of course, why?

Imposter Syndrome is a reaction to a set of circumstances, unrealistic self-expectation and/or stress which increases doubt in your abilities and can often explain the feeling of being a fraud or being 'caught out' somehow. It disproportionately affects high-achieving people (read women), who find it difficult to accept their accomplishments.[*] Many question whether they're deserving of accolades, doubt their abilities and feel like frauds at work. This is perpetrated through societal norms mostly seen in relationships and working environments.[†] It's a heavy load to bear, but it's one of 'female-centred hysteria' that is forced upon us to fix. Before the term Imposter Syndrome became the norm, women were pushing against this diagnosis, and I want to see that strength resurge again.

So firstly, why women specifically? Blame is at the heart of Imposter Syndrome and is very much an individual infliction. A constant lack of physical representation is just one of the factors that feeds into Imposter Syndrome. For instance, pervasive racist and sexist stereotypes can cause marginalised people to doubt themselves. When

---

[*] APA.org, https://www.apa.org/gradpsych/2013/11/fraud
[†] *Harvard Business Review*, 'Stop Telling Women They Have Imposter Syndrome'

Imposter Syndrome is often diagnosed on a woman, it neglects to account for systemic bias, classism, xenophobia and exclusion, which is always worth discussing. Women think feeling like an outsider is an illusion, but it isn't. It, like many other systems we are forced to accept as a way of life, was specifically made this way to keep the order of things complimentary for a select few. In the workplace specifically, progression is a pathologised tactic to keep certain figures in leadership roles and others in the more uncomfortable, laborious or tedious positions. Questioning this? Look at your leadership and those who are on average promoted more than others. See any similarities or notice-able characteristics? Yeah. That part. 75% of senior level corporate women report having personally experienced Imposter Syndrome at certain points in their career and 81% believe they put more pressure on themselves not to fail than men do.*

So how does this specifically affect Black women, and why? As Black women, we are told often that our voices aren't loud enough and that we have to work twice as hard. Add to that that we are the most endangered of the human race and are often left undefended. No matter how well intentioned these comments and sharing of infographics are, we are not just statistics, we are people and this lens is heavy to hold and exist through. As a Black woman, it's easy to feel like you're constantly left out of the equation, the pecking order, the hierarchy and even studies. The lack

* *Forbes*, 'Impostor Syndrome Prevalence In Professional Women And How To Overcome It'

of representation is guaranteed to make you feel inferior and excluded. Many of us across the world are implicitly, if not explicitly, told we don't belong in white- and male-dominated workplaces. Many Black women leave or lose their jobs, while citing feelings of marginalisation or disillusionment, which is consistent with our experiences across the board. Even in some of the biggest phenomenon's of our generation and recent times, the great resignation or quiet quitting movement, it's more complicated for us to be a part of this and the complexities stretch from being overly micromanaged in the first place, to being unrecognised in the workplace to disproportionate backlash from companies specifically for Black employees. It's historic too – severe forms of backlash including beatings, ridicule and death are what we know to be the norm, in part due to the experiences during and after transatlantic slave trade.* From 2018, there's been a shift and these experiences, plus feelings of exacerbated self-doubt, were key reasons why we as Black women began to make our transitions from corporate workplaces to entrepreneurship and scaling side hustles over the last few years. There is a movement happening (by us) within a movement not made for us. As for the lack of representation, that time is coming to a swift end! There was a time we weren't represented in beauty campaigns, in the media, but thanks to Web2 (the current internet format) and social media we've made our own safe

---

* *Insider*, '"Quiet quitting is not for us": Black employees share why quiet quitting is not for people of color — and why they're outright quitting instead'

spaces, communities and more importantly, we've owned our images and rights to content that represents us so well, we've made a clear path for visibility of the Black female in a narrative we relate to best. While we may not have it all yet, we have ownership over ourselves to some degree. Maybe one day very soon we can say 'as a Black woman, we can have it all' and have multiple sources to prove it. We need more of this. Let's hope Web3 will be that media change we need to bend the pendulum again.

> **Fun fact:** Some of our favourite Black icons including Supreme Court Justice Ketanji Brown Jackson, NASA engineer Maureen Zappala, actress Viola Davis and the former First Lady Michelle Obama have confessed to experiencing Imposter Syndrome.

After saying all that, it feels cruel to then admit that it's also a total beast to overcome. Sometimes no matter what you achieve or who you get cosigns and support from, you may still hear that tiny little voice in the back of your head telling you it's a fluke and the success won't last. And while there's currently no cure for it (though I'll keep you all posted), there are techniques that we can grasp on to make sure it doesn't hold the power to jeopardise our lives. Keep referring to these when you feel the pangs coming on.

And remember, Imposter Syndrome is not a 'you' or a 'female' issue. It's especially prevalent in biased and toxic cultures that value individualism and overwork. Aim to fix the bias, not the woman.

WAYS TO COMBAT IMPOSTER SYNDROME

See the signs. This first step is an oldie but a goodie. Naming the things you're going through is so often taken for granted but the catharsis of it can't be understated. Even if you tell one person and that one person is actually just your journal, taking the time to intentionally acknowledge that not all the things your brain tells you are 100% fact can be the first step to lowering the volume just that little bit!

- Feeling unsure doesn't make you an imposter – it's a feeling and not a fact.
- Track your wins. Another great way to gather the indisputable evidence *against* the claim that you are inexperienced or undeserving is to quite literally run the stats every once in a while. Think about the things you're most proud of doing this year or your favourite bucket list moments and write them down every time you're feeling wobbly about life. Alternatively, take a few minutes to compile a master list of all of the great and beautiful things you've done in your life, sprinkle a few doodles in there and plaster that baby to the wall for all to see. It can serve as a reminder in those shaky times that the rumours are not in fact true, and you are categorically, that bitch. By no means does the list need to be centred around a job either, you could have killed it in your Year Nine talent show or done an incredible job helping raise your baby sister. Maybe you're the best at

cooking jollof in the house or you swear you once beat Usain Bolt's time in the 100 metres on Sports Day that one year – think of the things that make you shine to you and you alone and allow yourself to luxuriate in them from time to time.

- **Talk to someone.** A theme that's recurring throughout this book is the power of communication. I think it's something we all understand deep in our core, but for some reason, it's harder for some of us to accept and act on. Be it getting involved in a mentorship scheme where you can bounce these anxieties off of someone who will almost definitely have been there, speaking to your boss at work and floating the idea of leadership or management training to help combat it, telling your parents about the doubts you're having or seeking professional help from a therapist, talking to someone can be invaluable. As scary as it feels to take that leap into vulnerability, the rewards of a supportive ear and a second opinion can often be a huge help to snap you out of a negative spiral and view yourself through the kind eyes of another.

- **Tame the beast.** Okay now, this last tip is a bit of a rogue one and may not be approved by a licensed professional, but here we go anyway. I think one of the ways to overcome Imposter Syndrome is to embrace the things that it gives you. Stay with me. It's not ideal by any means, but one of the ways that I found a lot of comfort on my own journey with anxiety was taking a second to reflect on the ways in which it's made me who I am today and the things that I've achieved because of that person. What I mean by that is, maybe you had a job interview and despite you being entirely qualified, you were so intent on meticulously preparing for every worst-case scenario that you were the most organised and compelling candidate for the job. Maybe your Imposter Syndrome means that you have a level of empathy for those who are struggling and can use that to help bring new voices and people into your own industry. Maybe dealing with Imposter Syndrome means that you see the signs of it in someone else and are able to hold space for each other in a professional setting. It's not necessarily a sustainable long-term fix and Imposter Syndrome is still an innately stressful and unpleasant experience, but being able to see and embrace its small positive impact on you can be a way of helping you get through the worst times.

- **Challenge negative self-talk.** Stay attuned to vague self-deprecating comments such as: 'I am so stupid!', 'I can't do presentations!' or 'I have no business being in this job or position!' In these moments, stick with the facts, stay focused and work to create distance between the evidence and your self-statements.

- **Counteract the stereotypes.** Remind yourself that key tasks and performance are not and have never been affected by gender or race. The idea that they are affected by gender or race is a lie perpetuated by an intention to keep us and others like us in our place. I say, 'bun that – respectfully'.

Now that we've kicked Imposter Syndrome's ass, I guess we can talk a bit more about ways we can speak up for ourselves and advocate for the things that we know we deserve.

The first context I always think is tricky to toe the line in is professional settings. And within that, I think pay is a great place to start. I don't know whether it's years of unequal pay or feeling underestimated, but I've come to the conclusion that, at this point, it's easiest to assume that as a Black woman living life in this UK, 99.9% of the time whatever I am being offered as financial compensation for a job is absolutely not the maximum of what a company is able to pay me from the work. I can probably count on my hands the number of times I have been offered an amount, asked for more and it has *genuinely* transpired that the person was being fully transparent about the budget limitations with their initial offer. And I find that super depressing.

Just the other day, I saw a TikTok video concentrating on one word that this creator believed can tip the scales when it comes to any kind of negotiation. A word that can tip the balance of power into situations that can often feel super nerve-wracking and unequal. That word is 'fair'. This creator (@digitaltalentmanager) points out how the subtle phrasing introduces this idea of value exchange – that in a negotiation you're not only trying to gain from the other person but you're also trying to give them something too. A perfect example of this would be when you're in conversations about a pay rise at work that's overdue but you're facing some resistance. Chances are you're not sitting there in that office asking for free money with no justification or founding. You're negotiating a deal that is supposed to represent the added value that you contribute to the company through years of expertise and experience in your field and the pay rise or promotion will undoubtedly come with a collection of added responsibilities and requirements from you as an employee, too. Being able to reframe that request as a fair and reasonable one removes any crumbs of that doubt that you aren't deserving of what you're asking for or that your place of work is somehow doing you a favour, when in fact the agreement is something that benefits you both. It's a small but mighty mindset shift that can help you erase that whispering guilt that your wins are somehow flukes or that your growth and progression professionally is just something that you're 'getting away with'.

BOUNDARY SETTING

I think one of the most crucial and often hard parts of self-advocacy can be setting boundaries. For those of us who are ambitious or motivated, there's an ease that comes with knowing what you might want out of a situation. Setting goals can feel intimidating but at least they make what we are aiming for clearer in our own minds as we move through life. Boundaries on the other hand can feel a little scary. With boundaries come 'no's and with 'no's come rejection and worse-case scenarios. 'What if another opportunity doesn't come around?' 'What if they find someone else?' 'What if they don't want to work with me again?' And I'm not going to lie, these are all valid questions! But when it comes to tackling wellness and creating the most supportive environment for personal and professional growth, the answer simply has to be that the honouring of the boundary you've set has to come before the job, the gig, the title, because we shouldn't have to occupy spaces or perform tasks that don't respect those boundaries in the first place. If a company comes to you on a Friday afternoon with a project that they want completed by Monday morning and one of your boundaries is that your weekends are your dedicated downtime, then that's what I'd call a match made in hell. No matter how incredible the opportunity might be, it's blatantly clear from the offset that you and this company's ways of operating are in direct opposition with each other. And while your anxious mind might be telling you that you should be terrified of turning it down, maybe it even says something like, 'it's a good opportunity so just say yes this time and then next time . . .', there really is no better time to assert yourself than the present. Boundaries pushed once will only continue to recede, and if anything, they'll become even harder to enforce over time, because the precedent has already been set!

Often the fear that you can feel when asking for more or passing on an opportunity stems from something called a *scarcity mindset* – the idea that resources are not only limited but there also aren't enough of them to go around. It's a philosophy that can often spark feelings of competition, jealousy and insecurity, because if there's not enough out there for all of us to eat, then … let the Hunger Games begin. But whether it's related to jobs, money, attention, partners, whatever it might be – living in a state of constant threat and fear is not a healthy space to exist in. Instead, a reassuring perspective that I always try to counteract my fight-or-flight reflexes with is the *abundance mindset*. Because for every force there is an equal and opposite force!

The abundance mindset is fairly self-explanatory in that it's really just the belief that there is *always* enough to go around. Enough success, enough joy, enough love, enough attention, enough opportunity. It's something that you have to remind yourself of whenever you feel threatened by someone else's wins or when you feel disempowered to ask for exactly what you want. The thinking is that, if there's enough to go around and I have a certain list of requirements, then by advocating for myself and asking for them, either I will be denied what I have requested and something better and more suited to me will inevitably come along, or what I ask for is perfectly reasonable and my needs will be met. Win–win. Some of the other ways that the abundance mindset can really elevate the way you navigate professional spaces is that it allows us to view our own peers through a vastly more positive light, because they are no longer our competition but instead they're our comrades. And what do you do with comrades? You help each other out, you collaborate, you share information, and you learn to think bigger.

Don't get me wrong, I'm aware that taking that kind of position comes from a place of privilege too – the privilege to go without in the moment if need be. But setting boundaries isn't always as cut and dried as you'd think, it doesn't always have to be an absolute yes or an absolute no. Sometimes setting boundaries is just as simple as knowing what it is you need to perform at your best and making sure you put structures in place that help you maintain that. If you work a super-intense job with mammoth hours and have other responsibilities in your personal life, maybe you can't do emails after 4:59 p.m., or tell your boss you need flexible WFH hours. But instead, it's essential that you carve out one evening a week to devote entirely to a passion project that you can indulge in and enjoy alone with no pressure or end goal. If your job requires you to work long hours, maybe you concede a little more of your weekday evenings, but your weekends become your sacred space. Or you make sure you take every last one of your entitled leave days and partake in some radical rest somewhere far far away.

The first step in setting boundaries is identifying precisely where your limits lie in the first place. A tip is to look out for patterns of what makes you tense, uncomfortable, frustrated, resentful or withdrawn. That could manifest in big or small ways like you getting quiet in a meeting, needing to take a walk, always procrastinating over the same activities, needing a cathartic release or feeling the physiological symptoms of anxiety. Once you've taken note of those, it's good to figure out what exactly you'd like to or can be changed about the way things are currently working out. That's where your own knowledge about the realms of possibility and context really come into play. What would a better or more ideal situation look like? Have you seen it happen before? Does it make sense and is it justifiable? Once you've assessed that, the next step is all about communication, a relatively loaded dice in professional spaces but also a place where clear and well-documented communication can play to your advantage. Take the time to really craft and finesse your wording, get a friend to look it over if you have to, re-read it, sit with it for a while, and most importantly, avoid sending it in moments when your emotions are already heightened.

Some other pointers would be to use language that opens up the dialogue between you and the person you're speaking to – to show that you're open to hear their perspective as well. Try not to get defensive, but also communicate assertively so that it's clear what you're asking for. Avoid language that has accusatory structures or feels like a complaint without a constructive angle, focus on statements that specifically pertain to you, 'I believe that . . .', 'I would . . .' Executive coach and author Melody Wilding has an incredible full suite of resources that break down the importance and formation of boundaries too, if you're ever looking to dig deeper into how and why we form them.

The last thing I will say about boundary-setting is that it's not just worth doing when it's a resounding success. There's a chance that when setting your boundaries, you are going to be met with flared-up, emotional responses, resistance or even gaslighting. When entering a situation, it's super useful to spitball some potential responses to these kinds of scenarios. But even more importantly than that, you have to remember that the most revolutionary part lies in the act of setting the boundary – that's the bit that you control and are responsible for. What you're not responsible for is what other people do with the boundaries that you set and how they receive them.

All of that is on them. But the practice of listening to yourself, your needs and fighting to honour them is more than enough in the first place. And if you do so with the tools laid out, then what happens once those needs are out of your hands and in the hands of those you require them from, will make it clear exactly what you need to do next.

> 'To me, Black feminism is strength in knowing who you are, what you want, what you deserve and not wavering when people try to tell you otherwise. Standing in the core of that.'
> – Char Ellesse

ADVOCATE IN RELATIONSHIPS

When it comes to self-advocacy within personal relationships, there are definitely some similarities and differences when you compare it to advocating for yourself in the workplace. I think that ultimate takeaway rings true in most interpersonal scenarios, too. The act of self-advocacy with your partner or your friend in a healthy, open and empathetic way is the part that you can control and take accountability for. What that person decides to do with your communication is entirely a reflection of them in that situation. And if they show you who they really are once you've taken those measures, then it's once again up to you to decide where your own boundaries lie and what you're willing to accept. I think the process for unpacking your boundaries is fairly similar. Follow the red flags of discomfort when you spend time with them and interrogate what could help alleviate some of that tension and stress for you.

But when it comes to how you communicate those boundaries with them and the directional nature of the exchange, I think that's where the two categories split apart. Your relation to your employer at its core is not just transactional but also hierarchical. You enter into an often literal but always metaphorical contract of the things that you are supposed to provide for each other and both have these more clear-cut frameworks to refer to and negotiate when opinions start to differ. Your social relationships with friends and the people you love generally are so much more blurred and fluid. There's a social contract that we all implicitly abide by just by existing within our society, but you don't purely occupy any one single role even in one single relationship. To your partner you could one day be the therapist's ear, the next you are a provider and the next they aren't reliant on you at all, and vice versa. As a result, the relationship and the ways that you go about setting boundaries with them need to reflect the more flexible, equal and symbiotic relationship that you have. Where you have your boundaries, they will also have theirs which are equally valid. And where negotiation and compromise are things you can make a call on whether you're willing to use them in a job salary discussion, unless you're planning to walk away from your partner entirely, your boundary-setting will be more of a give-and-take discussion.

At the same time of course, I have to add that we do all have dealbreaker boundaries in relationships and those are crucial to establish super early on. Once those are broken or challenged, you are absolutely well within your rights to walk away. Dealbreaker boundaries can look like: discussing or being able to confidently discuss and define your future(s) – e.g. thoughts on marriage, children, family, religious practices, living standards and goals as well as your financial stability and hopes, trust, respect for boundaries, conflict and the way its handled, abuse, codependency, comfortability around each other and self-centred attitudes.

It's important to know your triggers both in this sense and also in the sense of those softer boundaries that you might have that aren't fatal but you want to pay attention to. Constant communication and interrogation of these will help you ensure that there's no assumed knowledge that your partner will 'just know' what you are and are not comfortable with unless you tell them. It'll also ensure that you can find and embed your own coping mechanisms for spotting what upsets you and finding ways to heal from that alongside whatever boundaries you set with your partner to be sensitive of. For example, if I was disgusted by the sight of a banana and every time I saw one it just set me off, that's something I should absolutely flag as a potential hiccup in my relationship. I might say, 'I really hate bananas; they make me feel unsafe.' I may even have to remind my partner a couple of times if it's something that's pretty specific to me

185

or they haven't come across something similar before. But after a while, I'd expect their behaviour to shift to accommodate that boundary that I have – whether that looks like a universal banana embargo in our house at all times or just an effort made not to eat them when I'm anywhere in the vicinity. Even if they quite like bananas. Simultaneously, however, I would also (hopefully) take it upon myself to start to unpick and reconcile this quality within myself too. Why *do* bananas make me feel so unsafe? Did something happen with them in my childhood that I've blocked out? Is it part of a more deep-rooted issue? How can I make sure that I'm also doing the work to not surrender to every phobia I have and instead am making strides to meet my banana-loving partner in the middle of this so that we both have a good quality of life? I realise I've drawn the banana analogy all the way out now, and I apologise for that but hopefully the point is clear.

When it comes to setting boundaries with friends, family and partners, I also think it's really key to express the love that you have for them alongside the requests you might be making. Seeing them as the human beings that they are, just as flawed as you, and reassuring them that your boundaries are not an attack on them or their character (unless they actually are, lol). But in most cases, taking the time and effort to actually communicate the things you want out of a relationship isn't taken as the act of love that it really is and reinforcing the value you appreciate in them is one way to do that more obviously. Ultimately, advocating for yourself in any kind of relationship is a way of saying that you value the connection so much that you actively want to work to make it the best that it can be. Rather than throwing in the towel or taking those more short-term reactionary or knee-jerk responses, you are hopeful and believe that you can move and grow past the issues you have and the process of that will be worth it. And is there any clearer declaration of love and commitment than that, really?

> 'If we don't fight for ourselves, nobody's fighting for us.'
> – Char Ellesse

MEDICAL ADVOCACY

Medical advocacy can often feel like the scariest kind of advocacy because so many of us feel out of our depth when it comes to the world of medicine with all its terms and long-ass names. To think that the people whose hands we place our lives in, that have spent years of their lives and thousands of pounds on training for these professions, might be just as fallible as us is frankly terrifying. But it's also the truth. And in a world where prejudices and flat-out racism are still massively prevalent, I hate to break it to you but there isn't one single doctor on this planet that was brought up in a vacuum. What that means is that bias skews the perspectives of human beings in every profession from policing to journalism to tech, and this means the same bias is categorically bound to leak into all corners of medicine too. And the stats back it up, too. Black women are *four times more likely* to die in pregnancy and childbirth, according to a report released in 2021 by MBRRACE-UK. Roughly the same horrific numbers apply over in the States too.* And to be clear, the disparity can't be linked to one overarching health condition that we're predisposed to that's fatal or incurable. We're at risk of broadly the same complications as our white counterparts, but for some reason in the hands of trusted medical professionals, we are not making it out of these rooms unharmed anywhere near as often.

And this is the reason why medical advocacy is absolutely imperative for our survival and for the wellbeing of the next generation of us who suffer these losses as well. When Serena Williams spoke out about her pregnancy complications it really hit home for me that this issue is so much bigger than any one person, or something that money can buy your way out of even. But at least if we come armed with the strategy to fight for our own lives, maybe we can save them. And this extends far beyond pregnancy too. Each person's healthy journey is so personal and varied, but I hope this little checklist I put together can act as a 101 on medical advocacy regardless of the concerns you're coming with.

1. Book an appointment. For starters: if in doubt, please just book it. I know that I for one have fallen at that first hurdle enough times. Especially with the NHS operating in the end times, it can feel

---

* birthrights.org.uk, 'New MBRRACE report shows Black women still four times more likely to die in pregnancy and childbirth'

like a burden to prioritise your own health, but I cannot say it enough: BOOK THE APPOINT-MENT, FRIEND. And when you do, be sure to think about and then explain exactly what it is you're looking to get out of it to yourself, to the receptionist, to the doctor, even to your dog (if that helps you practise).

2. Come prepared. This doesn't mean print off that worst-case scenario from WebMD, but it means doing some actual research. It sucks that it has to come to this, but you'd rather have the knowledge and options that seem most viable to you before-hand so that you're able to make sure nothing gets missed or ruled out prematurely. The second layer of that preparation can feel like overkill, but it's to also come prepared for the event that you get stage fright too: a notebook with the key points you want to discuss that you can also use to take new notes from the appointment to refer back to later.

3. Don't be afraid to ask questions. That's literally what they are there for, even if they roll their eyes at you. Ask all the questions that pop into your head to make sure that you utilise that face-to-face time, and if they say something you don't under-stand, don't you dare feel too ashamed to ask for clarification! Some of these man have been doing these jobs since before the internet was invented and still get it wrong, don't let them make you feel less than for needing clarity.

4. Keep your own records. When you take notes, ensure you keep them in one place, dated and make them as comprehensive as possible. It's a great way to hold your doctor accountable if and when you face resistance, are referred, want to change GPs or do further research. Take note of symptoms as and when they occur too so that you feel as confident in the accuracy of your account as you possibly can. Sadly, this sometimes also helps the doctors believe you more, which is total nonsense, I know.

5. Shop around. I know doctors hate this, but in every way that counts, it's literally not about them. Never hesitate to get a second opinion when it comes to serious health concerns or diagnosis. There's literally no worse-case scenario. Either they confirm what's been established and you feel more confident in it, or they don't and know you have that information too.

6. Bring backup. This one needs to be charged to the game because as soul-destroying as it can be, sometimes we just have to acknowledge how messed up the world can be and make the moves accordingly. If you have the option to bring support with you when being treated or seen by a doctor, please go ahead and do that. And do not let them make you feel bad for doing so. They don't even need to contribute, sometimes it can just be good to apply pressure with a witness, and when appointments are overwhelming, that's one more

person to take notes and process the information on your behalf too.

7. **Trust your gut.** The last one feels a bit wishy washy but given the circumstances I think it needs to be said. Always listen to your body. You are the person who spends every second with it, who knows it inside out and can feel what it is to live inside it. No one will be a better judge of the shift within it than you are, no matter what they tell you. If something doesn't feel right, say it. If you notice a weird pattern between your meds and a side effect, say it. If nothing feels like it's working, speak up and say it. Literally, what is the worst that could happen?

Eleven

MAKING A CHANGE

I wanted to take this chapter to acknowledge the difficulty in actually making the change that we want to see both in ourselves and out in the world too. It's all well and good talking about all the things we want in life and all the ways that we could be and do better, but we have to remember that at the same time we're also creatures of habit. And in order to break patterns and routines that we've lived with for our entire lives, we first have to realise just how deep they run and how hard it can be. Otherwise, you can end up living in this really tedious limbo between the person you are today and the person you want to be, where it feels like if it doesn't happen instantly it might never. But I promise you that's not true. Real, deep, meaningful change is not an overnight transformation or life makeover; it's small and deliberate everyday decisions and battles to move forward instead of staying stuck.

So, I've put together some of the most helpful tools I've employed over the years for inspiring change within myself and making strides towards my goals.

THERAPY

What I'm about to suggest here is an idea that I'm sure you've already flirted with or considered for yourself if you're sitting here reading this book, to be honest. And I'm not so deluded that I think this recommendation from me alone would be enough to convince you if you haven't already delved in at this point. But what I will say is that there is no greater tool than therapy for looking back at your past, assessing your behaviour, the causes of it, how it manifests in your life today and trying to find a way through it. That's quite literally what it was designed for. Because of the world we live in, it's not the easiest resource in the world to get a hold of, but if you have the means or some time to join the back of the queue, I really cannot recommend it enough as a way to gain a new and more constructive perspective on life outside of your own emotions and impulses. For those who are scared of what it might unearth, I hear you and I was definitely one of you when I first started. Therapy requires clearing significant mental space and time in your life to process what it digs up and to overcome it, and with the hectic lives so many of us are living, that can feel like a really tall order. But what I will say is that the effort it takes to dredge up these heavy conversations now becomes an equal and opposite lightness in the long term. Once you're armed with the knowledge and the tools to reflect on and retrain your behaviour into healthy patterns and actions, literally anything is possible!

If, on the other hand, you've ever considered therapy as

something that might not work for you because you don't feel like your situation is 'bad enough' or at crisis point ... sis, I'm here to tell you – no, *urge* you – if therapy is something that you think could benefit you in even the smallest of ways, please take the action before disaster strikes. Yes, therapy can be an incredibly effective way to pull you back from the brink when you are seriously struggling, but it can also be preventative and arm you with techniques to stop it from ever even getting there. I think we have this cartoonish image of someone who is 'broken' weeping on a leather couch while an old white lady observes with her legs crossed and writes furiously in her notepad. In reality, however, I really think we should all have a space that we can go to on a weekly basis and speak about whatever is weighing on our heart to an empathetic and objective listener who literally gets paid for the emotional labour they are undertaking. In fact, it's kind of mad to me that it's not mandatory.

And don't get it twisted, it may not always feel like the release that it will be in the long run. The first person you try could be a total wrong fit and not pass the vibe check. It could take a month before you feel like you've even scratched the surface. But even in the act of beginning that soul-searching and reflection is where the magic starts to happen, unlocking a new gaze that extends far beyond the 50 minutes you pay for and into your day-to-day, one of awareness, of questioning, even of straightforward curiosity about yourself as this complex and beautiful being that has been through so much and overcome a ton, but still has so much to learn.

So yeah, before I preach on for too long about it and bore you, take this as your sign if you've been agnostic about making that phone call or sending that enquiry email. It won't be an instant change, but it is one of the best investments of time and money that you can possibly make in yourself.

For an incredible resource that might push you that one step closer to investing in therapy and discovering different forms of therapy and which types might be well suited to your needs, please visit https://therapyforblackgirls.com.

VISION-BOARDING

This next method of inspiring inner change is a slightly controversial one. Talk to the wrong person about it and you may just be met with an eye roll and a dismissive hand wave. But in the eyes of those who are open to the possibilities and believe in the value of visualisation and manifestation? Vision boards are like the holy text. Part of the beauty of them is that they really do come in all different shapes and sizes, both analogue and digital. You could be of the traditional magazine cut-out school of thought or more of a Pinterest or Canva bandit, but whatever way you slice it, there is definitely a very real and tangible benefit to being able to physically see the change that you would like to enact right in front of you on a regular basis.

The practice of curating your vision board alone to balance your ambitions for love, life, your family, friends, career and health is something that we so rarely make the time to do, despite it forming the fuel for everything we do in our lives. I think taking the time at least twice a year (some make it a new year's tradition, others do it more seasonally) to check in with yourself about your priorities and desires is the perfect way to boost motivation, inspire change and feel a renewed sense of purpose. Find the perfect image that speaks to you for any given section and ask yourself why it does. Identify the aspects you'd like to apply to your own life and have a think about some of the steps you could take to get yourself there.

Thinking retrospectively too, vision boards also become a beautiful archive of all the dreams you've had over the years that you've either achieved, have stayed with you or you've let go of in replacement of new dreams. For my more seasoned vision-boarders out there, it can be such a trip to look back over years of manifestations and chart your growth, not just through your achievements but also in terms of the things you centred within your life from then to now. How and why have your sights shifted? Are there any lessons you've learnt that inform your dreams today? Things you wish you'd known back then that you know now?

GOAL-SETTING

Goal-setting can seem like a super-straightforward task but there are actually a lot of different techniques to help make the process as effective and intentional as possible in order to not just list out words on paper but also break down the real-life meaning of them and inspire the motivation to act on them too.

One method, developed by clinical psychologists William R. Miller and Stephen Rollnick, is called 'motivational interviewing'. It's a form of counselling and questioning that interrogates the drive behind the change we want to make and uses it to energise and strengthen our intentions to make them with open-ended questions, acceptance and collaboration. The result is something called 'change talk', which is fitting. It's that very dialogue that this book is all about, how we shift and grow as people over time.

Start by identifying the thing that you would like to change. It could be something broad like 'I'm bad at communicating' or something as simple as 'I go to bed too late' – what are the areas of your life that you would most like to change at this moment in time? After that, try to roughly prioritise them in terms of those that feel like the most pressing versus those that are smaller and less important. It doesn't have to be that the biggest problem is the most important problem for you. Maybe your largest issue is less relevant right now because you're currently single so it doesn't have an outlet to manifest, and what is really impacting the quality of your everyday life is actually not getting to bed until 3 a.m. and then waking up at 7 a.m. Think about *you* specifically and what you care about.

Next up, it's really important to wrap your head around the real motivation behind the change you want to effect. Why is it important to you to communicate better or to sleep more? What will change for the better if you're able to remedy this? This could be a list of things: e.g. my friendships will become more fruitful, I will feel more heard and seen, someone might be able to help me with the problems I'm facing, I'll feel less alone. I think this step is super key not just because it grounds our goals in a better future that we can then envisage (and can maybe even slap up on our vision board, eh?) but also because it helps bring to light the transformative power of the goals we have and, perhaps contrastingly, those that are based more in self-critique too. I am guilty time and time again of listing out all the ways I could change and be a different person, particularly when I'm in a negative slump. Some of the things I wish I could 'fix' are genuine concerns, but other times it's just me letting negative self-talk get in the way of appreciating myself as the person that I am. These toxic ideas that once I do X (like get a six-pack or drop a dress size or cop a certain jacket or pull off a certain hairstyle) then I'll be happy. Then everything will be fine. Then that trivial achievement will have such a positive impact on my life that at least all my problems will feel less big. But when you dig deeper it's just a mirage. Because when we centre these small goals that don't really reach the more deep-rooted issues and can't really change our life for the better in a substantial way, the goalposts keep on changing. There's always something else. By forcing ourselves to really analyse the transformative power of our goals before we make them our entire personality, we save ourselves YEARS of having to learn that lesson again and again.

After you've identified the motivation for the change you want to make, it's important to acknowledge the reality of where you are now. This is where the human psyche likes to play games, because if the difference between the reality and your ideal self is too small, it's hard to motivate yourself to do the work to make the change. But on the other hand, if the difference feels too vast, that can paralyse you too because you become demoralised. Making sure the goals you set yourself fall somewhere in the sweet spot between those two extremes is really key to feeling inspired and capable of making the changes you want to make.

Those parts are my favourite part of the theory, but there are also more exercises you can do to build that out for goals that you find particularly difficult to grasp too. More than anything though, don't be hard on yourself; sometimes you will let the goals slip. Whenever I would complain to my mum about not doing enough to commit to my goal, she would always tell me that you have to be okay with life happening and things slipping. So, if you're having a really difficult week at work, you might not have the energy to eat healthy or go to the gym – and that's fine! Acknowledge the slip and get back on track when you can. Remember life isn't a linear track upwards, instead it's ups, downs, bumps, obstacles. The journey takes unexpected turns, and so your goals might as well – it's best to embrace that than beat yourself up about it.

LITTLE BY LITTLE

By its very nature, change is intimidating as hell. It's the opposite of what we're wired to find comfortable, aka things that are consistent, predictable and known to us. The next step is pretty much the only way to make change in your life without causing a system error. When it comes to making goals, the best way is to start with the smallest shift possible.

Using the example of weight here purely because it's numerical, if your goal is to lose 10kg and that's all you envisage as you try to change up your diet, lifestyle and entire relation to the thing you do every day, the goal is going to seem so far from your reach that your brain will think it's completely abstract or just far too hard to do. With that same analogy, the things that you need to do to make the changes that will lead to that ultimate goal aren't as extreme as they might seem initially. They could be as small as the decision to put your exercise clothes at the foot of your bed before you go to sleep so that it's easier to motivate yourself to go to the gym in the morning. Or seeing that snack you love in the supermarket and counting to 10, closing your eyes and running away from it as fast as you can, lol. By the time you're at the checkout, there's nothing you can do about it . . . *insert Roll Safe meme*

But in all seriousness, applying that same theory to the more holistic goals that we might hold close to our hearts, the best way to visualise them and how we can get to them is to break them down into bite-size pieces that are far more digestible than the idea of an instant transformation. I want to succeed professionally as an X. To get there I need experience in X field first and to get that experience I need to either find a connection, network or show some kind of intention to enter that professional space. An example of that might be by starting your own blog, posting about your interests online or going for a coffee with one person whose career inspires you. And today that might just look like finding three people that could be good potential options for that and shooting off an email.

I find that the more specific and achievable my first few steps are, the easier I start to adjust, the more rewarding it feels and the more energy I'm able to generate to keep going further and further. Start as small as you feel is necessary; nothing's too embarrassing. If sending three emails gives you acid reflux, send one. If emails make you want to hurl, follow them on Instagram or LinkedIn or Twitter until you build the courage.

A POSITIVE IMPACT

Making change isn't just about the personal. Most of us would like to effect change in the world around us and make a difference to other people's lives. It's a great thing to try and make a positive impact in the lives of others and it's something that can build understanding, empathetic communities that stand up for each other. When issues build up to impact us as a community, I have always loved the way that we come together to push for change. In the Black community, we have always led the way when it comes to igniting and fighting for a different way of doing things. The civil rights movement, the #MeToo movement, the LGBTQIA+ movement – at the core of so many of these movements were Black people and people of colour tired of being treated as lesser than and ready to effect change no matter the cost.

Making A Change

Grassroots action is still so important in our communities, especially as so many issues in the world disproportionately affect us. A good example is climate change. Climate change is a real and pressing issue happening right now, negatively impacting Black and indigenous people and threatening their quality of life due to historic injustices. Thankfully, there are incredible people in the community speaking out to get their stories heard by those who have the power to turn the tide of climate change, namely Mikaela Loach and Elizabeth Yeampierre. Raising awareness for our plights is key to making a change and will serve to create a better future for us all.

That being said, it's also not your responsibility to fight every single battle. Read that again. This world is overwhelming and the amount of information and news at our fingertips can make us feel that every single issue in the world is ours to hold on to and to try and mend. This just can't be true. This planet is vast and we simply cannot understand or be advocates for every single person or community within it. As women, we can feel so much emotion and empathy for other people in the world going through things and that is a wonderful thing, but it can also lead to us suffering anxiety, depression and overwhelm. It's a brilliant thing to have empathy and it deserves to be channelled into something that will blossom from your attention. This might mean focusing more on issues in communities closer to home or taking the time to consider and research what causes might be currently underfunded and under-supported.

You making a change will look entirely different to

what someone else does, but doing something good simply because it will help people will have value no matter what package it comes in. You might volunteer at a foodbank every other week, you might donate to a charity once a month, you might be a part-time carer for a relative or you could be trying to make your workplace more inclusive and representative of the world. There are so many different options and opportunities to make a change outside of yourself and though it may not feel like a huge thing you are doing, little changes can add up to something unbelievable.

'Sometimes it is not always on you to be the person to speak, implement and ensure that [all] change is occurring. It's a domino effect and sometimes you are just one domino. It's about owning your part and doing what you can without feeling that you are responsible for the whole world.'
– Irene Agbontaen

SOCIAL MEDIA

By now this feels pretty obvious to say but, for all its downsides and biases, social media has also proved itself to be one of the greatest tools for change when creators and audiences choose to use it for good. It can raise awareness, help people feel less alone and bring traction to world issues that could have hardly been imagined pre-internet. Sadly, in the same breath, social media can spread misinformation about issues, it can encourage polarisation over uniting for change and it can make us feel like there is very rarely any good that happens in the world.

Social media is something that needs to be used carefully and with self-awareness. It is not the be-all and end-all to creating positive difference, and it certainly can have a great part to play in preventing change too. I don't want to tell you to delete all your social media accounts and remove yourself from it altogether, although it can be good to do that from time to time. If you are someone already completely off social media altogether, I get it, and just like we are covered with boundaries, this might be your personal boundary you need to live well.

If you are on social media, then you need to use it in a way that suits *you*. Not your followers, not the algorithm and not in a way you see others using it. You might lose followers for speaking up on issues that are important to you – does that mean you should stop? Absolutely not. Just as in life, you are not going to agree with everyone, and they may not agree with you. However, if we can be respectful and tolerant of those with differing opinions then we will create a safer space online. Be true to yourself and ensure you take time away from the platforms to have real conversations with real people. Not everything needs to be done online, especially if you don't have all the knowledge on the subject. Take a breath and stick that tweet in drafts if you need to.

Find balance where you can. Use it to promote your community, share your successes and failures (we could all do with being a bit more real about that), raise awareness for issues you feel passionately about and sometimes, be a

bit silly – not everything in life has to be serious. Sometimes making a change might mean being a bit more real,
a bit more of the weirdo you are and sharing that so other
people might feel more confident to embrace that side of
themselves. If it gets too much, step away. You exist in the
world, not online, so make sure you are nurturing yourself
beyond what you might be presenting online.

WELLNESS ACTION POINTS

1. **Make a list of your past successes.** We all have to
   get better at reflecting on and celebrating our past
   wins, because they contribute to where we are
   today and the place that we'll be coming from in
   the future too. Think about past versions of yourself
   that you've been and the changes and growth you've
   been able to make from then until now. What are
   some of the wins you're most proud of? How did
   they play into your strengths? What steps did you
   take to achieve them? Are there any lessons you
   could apply from those journeys or processes to
   the goals that you want to tackle moving forwards.
2. **Make a vision board.** Go on. I dare you. Make
   one and then tell me you don't feel like going out
   and conquering the whole entire world right that
   second. All the instructions are above so I won't
   repeat myself, but if you do make one inspired or
   reminded by this chapter, please feel free to tag
   me in it, so I can rejoice for you too ♥
3. **Set a date to check in with yourself.** Now I know

what you might be thinking and why this one might be getting your heart rate and blood pressure up, but hear me out. This date is not a deadline. It could be in three months, it could be in a year, it could be in five years' time. This date is like those check-in points in video games (gamers please close your ears now) – you know those rings that you go through that save your progress so that if you run out of XP or whatever? That's the point that you regenerate at and go from. I think when reading books like this or listening to podcasts like this or just in those moments where enough is enough and you feel the energy of 1,000 Red Bulls bursting through your veins, it can be really easy to harness that productivity and motivation in that moment and then forget about it when life gets busy again. Not because you no longer care but maybe you're just distracted or time got away with you a bit. Putting a reminder in your calendar or making it an anniversary-type affair just means that you are prompted to at the very least revisit where you were at the time and re-evaluate if your priorities are still the same or have changed drastically. It's not about getting yourself a gold sticker if you've achieved your goal (although that does sound adorable) or punishing yourself if you perceive that you've 'failed' or fallen short. Honestly, none of that is as important as the practice and habit of the actual self-reflection, and with time, you'll hopefully find that that embedded regularity actually helps to keep you honest and accountable to yourself because the concept of self-interrogation is no longer quite so scary or foreign to you.

4. Start saying yes. We've all seen the film *Yes Man* with Jim Carrey, right? If you haven't, consider this your cue to get on it. But either way, the sentiment is simple and effective. Making up excuses, giving things a pass, playing down our goals and doubting ourselves are such normalised and frankly natural behaviours of the world we live in that often we don't even notice we're doing them. In many ways, saying 'yes' is the smallest change you can make in any given moment. Especially if you send it via text ☺. Even thinking about the idea of making the conscious effort to rebalance your 'no' to 'yes' ratio can start a chain reaction of new experiences in your life that you would have otherwise missed out on. That coffee with an internet mutual that you know will make you a bit nervous because you can get awkward around strangers? Fuck it, what day's good for you? That hairstyle that you've had saved on your Pinterest for three years now but never had the courage to follow through with? Get auntie on the phone today because it's time. That job opportunity or commission that you're scared to accept because you think they picked the wrong person or you don't want to mess it up? It would quite literally be racist and sexist for you to decline. Sis, please

collect the bag. That yoga class that you're waiting for a friend to be available for to accompany you? Sis, the friend is not coming. You know it, I know it. Let's please both accept it and move on accordingly. I am challenging you to trial this challenge for just one week of saying yes to one thing that you would have otherwise found an excuse for, and see how, if nothing else, it shows you that even if we are in a simulation, we can still find ways to surprise ourselves at least.

Twelve

QUOTES TO REMEMBER & AFFIRMATIONS TO LIVE BY

There is always something so affirming and comforting about the words of others. They remind us of things we may have forgotten, they bolster us and rally us, they can even be transformative. I won't say my words in this book have been all *that* . . . but if they have, please feel free to write that five-star review, sis, lol.

Words are powerful, and so I wanted to dedicate a chapter of this book to highlighting some incredible quotes from people who have lived and learnt and thought deeply about life and our experiences. I also wanted to take a minute to acknowledge the power of your own words. Words of affirmation you write that are specific to you. Words that centre you.

QUOTES TO KEEP COMING BACK TO

'Anyone who's interested in making change in the world, also had to learn how to take care of herself, himself, theirselves.' – Angela Davis

Take Care

'Keep your eyes open' – Lashana Lynch

'The Dalai Lama teaches that we are all interconnected and inseparable from one another. Acknowledging that can make us less lonely, more compassionate and better investigators of the truth.' – Arthur C. Brooks

'I am deliberate and afraid of nothing.' – Audre Lorde

'Self-care is a vital component of self-preservation and survival.' – Dr Tiffany Lowe-Payne

'Two things can be true at once. You're allowed to feel weird and need something simultaneously. It's not either or.' – Nadine Bacchus

'It's not by mistake . . . it's not!' – Elsa Majimbo

'We need to do a better job of putting ourselves higher on our own to-do list.' – Michelle Obama

'What we do is more important than what we say or what we say we believe.' – bell hooks

'I'm convinced that we Black women possess a special indestructible strength that allows us to not only get down, but to get up, to get through, and to get over.' – Janet Jackson

'Freeing yourself was one thing; claiming ownership of that freed self was another.' – Toni Morrison

'You can't be hesitant about who you are.' – Viola Davis

Quotes To Remember & Affirmations To Live By

'Success is liking yourself, liking what you do and liking how you do it.' – Maya Angelou

'Any woman who wishes to be an intellectual, to write non-fiction, to deal with theory, faces a lot of discrimination coming her way, and perhaps even self-doubt, because there aren't that many who've gone before you. And I think that the most powerful tool we can have is to be clear about our intent. To know what it is we want to do rather than going into institutions thinking that the institution is going to frame for us.' – bell hooks

'You are your best thing.' – Toni Morrison

'I am a feminist, and what that means to me is much the same as the meaning of the fact that I am Black; it means that I must undertake to love myself and to respect myself as though my very life depends upon self-love and self-respect.' – June Jordan

'I always believed that when you follow your heart or your gut, when you really follow the things that feel great to you, you can never lose, because settling is the worst feeling in the world.' – Rihanna

'I realised that I don't have to be perfect. All I have to do is show up and enjoy the messy, imperfect and beautiful journey of my life.' – Kerry Washington

'Once we recognize what it is we are feeling, once we recognize we can feel deeply, love deeply, can feel joy, then we will demand that all parts of our lives produce that kind of joy.' – Audre Lorde

Take Care

'I have standards I don't plan on lowering for anybody . . . including myself.' – Zendaya

'Caring for myself is not self-indulgence; it is self-preservation, and that is an act of political warfare.' – Audre Lorde

'You've got to learn to leave the table when love's no longer being served.' – Nina Simone

'We have so much coming in as sisters, when is our interior life ever put at the forefront? We constantly want to give to other people . . . Too much of not caring for yourself is not a good thing. We're bad at that as achievers. Self-care is a priority and we have to do it more.' – Ava DuVernay

'Even if it makes others uncomfortable, I will love who I am.' – Janelle Monae

'Most of us did not learn when we were young that our capacity to be self-loving would be shaped by the work we do and whether that work enhances our wellbeing.' – bell hooks

'Never limit yourself because of others' limited imagination; never limit others because of your own limited imagination.' – Dr Mae Jemison

'If you are silent about your pain, they'll kill you and say you enjoyed it.' – Zora Neale Hurston

'I'm rooting for everybody Black.' – Issa Rae

Quotes To Remember & Affirmations To Live By

'If any female feels she need anything beyond herself to legitimate and validate her existence, she is already giving away her power to be self-defining, her agency.'
– bell hooks

'She can beat me, but she cannot beat my outfit.'
– Rihanna

'We are the ones we've been waiting for.' – June Jordan

'The most common way people give up their power is by thinking they don't have any.' – Alice Walker

'If we aren't intersectional, some of us, the most vulnerable, are going to fall through the cracks.'
– Kimberlé Williams Crenshaw

'I am here. I am whole. I am able.' – Alexandra Elle

'It's not the load that breaks you down; it's the way you carry it.' – Lena Horne

'When I dare to be powerful – to use my strength in the service of my vision, then it becomes less and less important whether I am afraid.' – Audre Lorde

'I really don't think life is about the I-could-have-beens. Life is only about the I-tried-to-do. I don't mind the failure, but I can't imagine that I'd forgive myself if I didn't try.'
– Nikki Giovanni

'I have a lot of things to prove to myself. One is that I can live my life fearlessly.' – Oprah Winfrey

Take Care

'A crown, if it hurts us, is not worth wearing.'
– Pearl Bailey

'You are on the eve of a complete victory. You can't go wrong. The world is behind you.' – Josephine Baker

'Don't wait around for other people to be happy for you. Any happiness you get you've got to make yourself.'
– Alice Walker

'As long as women are using class or race power to dominate other women, feminist sisterhood cannot be fully realized.'
– bell hooks

'My mission in life is not merely to survive, but to thrive; and to do so with some passion, some compassion, some humor, and some style.'
– Maya Angelou

'I'd rather regret the risks that didn't work out than the chances I didn't take at all.'
– Simone Biles

AFFIRMATIONS

I'm going to say something that might be illegal to say in a book, but I want you to highlight or underline three quotes that really hit you. The ones you read and went 'whew, if that ain't me'. Highlight them so you can go back to them and remember them and recite them. They might change their meaning to you over time but hold those words with you, because you never know, they might help you in a difficult time.

Affirmations are words for you, about you and by you. Affirmations are there to help you practise positive thinking and self-empowerment, because if you say it out loud, even if it feels weird, you are more likely to believe it. They can help you overcome your self-sabotaging, negative thoughts and they can build confidence over time. Your words should not be underestimated!

To get you started, I wanted to share a long list of some of my favourite affirmations of varying degrees of intensity and with different focuses. Choosing a few that you feel speak to you or an area that you'd like to focus your energy positively and finding subtle (or not so subtle!) ways to weave them into your daily life is a great way to encourage and support yourself and your goals, even if just subconsciously.

Whether that's writing a few down on Post-it notes for Future You to find on the fridge or in your bathroom medicine cabinet or using them on your mirror and taking five minutes to affirm them verbally to yourself while getting ready for the day or in a meditative moment. You could incorporate them into a piece of artwork that you set as your phone wallpaper, set them as reminders when you most need a boost in the day or dot them throughout your diary as a little pick-me-up to start your week intentionally.

I am abundant.

Take Care

What is meant for me, will find me.
Beautiful things are coming my way
and I cannot wait to greet them.

I am love, I am loving and I am loved.

I am a magnet for incredible opportunities and my
future is even brighter than I could possibly imagine.

My present is beautiful, and I feel lucky
and grateful to be here in this skin.

I am unique, I am valid and I am enough.

There is nothing I can't handle, and
nothing that is beyond my reach.

I do not compare myself to others, I love
myself exactly the way that I am.

I am precisely where I should be at this moment.

My triumphs are so much greater than my failures.

I accept what I cannot change and
change what I cannot accept.

I am powerful and beyond worthy of the greatness
I have and will continue to achieve.

Quotes To Remember & Affirmations To Live By

My mistakes do not define who I am.

I am doing my best and that is enough.

I accept and love myself unconditionally.

*The love that I have and provide for others
circles and returns to me infinitely.*

I give myself abundant space to grow and to learn.

I listen to my intuition and trust my gut.

*I accept myself fully for the person that I
am, and who I will be in the future.*

*I see and validate my emotions; I allow them
to exist fully and serve their purpose.*

*I give myself the care and attention
that I need and deserve.*

I am perfectly aligned with the energy of abundance.

I wholeheartedly believe in myself and my goals.

*My ambitions are limitless. All that I
desire is already in the making.*

I trust that I am on the right path.

Take Care

My mind is full of brilliant ideas.

I am creatively inspired by the world around me.

*I am gravitating closer to my truest
self with every passing day.*

I am worthy of all the good that life has to offer.

Healthy, vibrant energy flows through my body naturally.

*I welcome positive, healthy, blooming
energy with open arms.*

I breathe deeply and fully.

I make healthy choices and allow myself to thrive.

My body is always doing its best, I listen to its needs.

I am a magnet for good health.

I release myself from doubt and welcome faith.

*I am thankful for all that I have and
all that I will accomplish.*

I forgive myself and others.

Take some time to consider what affirmations might be
right for you and write down a couple now.

Thirteen

OUR SAYINGS

Black people across the world have always had sayings that are specific to our experiences and our lives. Often, these sayings aren't written down, and instead they remain in our collective consciousness through oral history. Our ancestors held wisdoms and understandings that deserve to be valued and held up as important words that can lead us to finding our truths. They can also be hilariously funny and wonderfully eclectic, as you'll see from the list I've pulled together below. From African tribes to the islands of the Caribbean, from the well-known to family-specific, these are sayings that have been created by us, for us. Feel free to add your own to this list, my hope is that we can make this book a record of our cultures and communities through the words they used to affirm themselves, teach lessons and reach down through history.

AFRICAN PROVERBS

'Only a fool tests the depth of a river with both feet.'

'[S]he who does not know one thing knows another.'

Take Care

'Do not look where you feel but where you slipped.'

'No matter how hot your anger is it cannot cook yams.'

'A roaring lion kills no game.'

'Teeth do not see poverty.'

'You have little power over what's not yours.'

'Where you will sit when you are old
shows where you stood in youth.'

'When the roots of a tree begin to decay,
it spreads death to the branches.'

'Birds sing not because they have answers
but because they have songs.'

'It is crooked wood that shows the best sculptor.'

'Be a mountain or lean on one.'

'Wisdom is like a baobab tree; no one
individual can embrace it.'

'If you are building a house and a nail breaks, do
you stop building or do you change the nail?'

'We want to give two things to our children. The
first one is roots; the other one is wings.'

'Family names are like flowers; they blossom in clusters.'

'Gold should be sold to the one
who knows the value of it.'

Our Sayings

*'If you are filled with pride then you
will have no room for wisdom.'*

THE CARIBBEAN

'Live and let live.' – The Pierre Family

'A nuh wan day monkey waan wife.' (Focus
on your future) – Jamaican proverb via The
Pierre Family and The Robinson Family

*'Hard is hard man. This is no more a tougher
journey than others.'* – Layla Lawson

'This too shall pass.' – Agnes Mwakatuma

'Let me tell you something.' – every Black woman ever

*'Every food is good to eat. Not everything
is good to say.'* – The Fanis Family

'Time will come, time will tell.' – The Pierre Family

*'Those who eat the meat, must suck the
bone.'* – St Lucian Proverb

'Chicken merry, hawk deh near.' (Don't get
too happy, something bad might happen.)
– Jamaican proverb via The Robinson Family

'Duppy know who fi frightin.' (Bullys know
who to pick on.) – Jamaican proverb
via The Robinson Family

Take Care

'If I ever lick you, you see how waata waak to a pumpkin belly.' (If I hit you, you'll be so stunned you'll understand the mysteries of life, for example, how water gets inside pumpkin.) – Jamaican proverb via The Robinson Family

'If trouble tek you, pickney shot (shirt) fit yuh.' (When you're in trouble adapt quickly to get out of it.) – Jamaican proverb via The Robinson Family

'Give him an inch, him tek a mile.' (You give people a chance and they take advantage of you.) – Jamaican proverb via The Robinson Family

'Wanti wanti cyaan get it.' (Stop watching what other people have and focus on your own life.) – Jamaican proverb via The Robinson Family

FURTHER ACROSS THE DIASPORA

'There's no such thing as better, just different.' – Shannie Mears

'When you are in the presence of wisdom, listen.' – Sheila Atim

'The ancestral energy is second to none.' – Lashana Lynch

'How dare we say we don't do enough. All we need is to be softer and kinder, to ourselves.' – Lashana Lynch

FINAL THOUGHTS

How would you summarise what you have read?

I said it at the beginning, but not only is this book for Black women, it is also conceptualised, written, proofed and contributed to by Black women and, most importantly, it is in support of Black women. Raising a toast and giving the most thanks to the ones who came before us, the ones here with us now and to the many who come after us. We are not in competition with each other; we are for each other.

I had some idea of how I might feel getting to the end, but nothing could prepare me for what it would actually be like. The reality is, I struggled during the process of this book – emotionally, physically, spiritually – but somehow, I held on, or rather this book and the opportunity held on to me, and thankfully because of that, I found myself again. I found myself in each of you reading it, in the contributor interviews, in the resources and, quite frankly, I'm in awe that even when I thought I was alone, I never was.

That is what being a Black woman means to me. It's more than strength; it's innate. It means to be completely real and transparent. To bring each other forward without burden or malice. I hope that sometime in the future, a Black woman can define herself and Black women as a whole as being free – free in spirit, free in our understanding, free of stereotypes, free to just be and exist however she wants and without confines or fear of abuse. This isn't just for the few; this needs to be for us all.

Writing a book for Black women, specifically in relation to our wellbeing, was no easy task, but it was therapeutic. As much as I wanted to keep writing and to try and cover every topic relevant to us (spoiler: there's just too many), I really couldn't do it all but I hope what I have done, what *we* have done, is just enough for us now and that we can build upon this guide, having reached a few wellbeing milestones personally and collectively alongside this book.

No doubt there were moments in this book that hit you hard and possibly times when not everything resonated and that's okay. Nevertheless, I want you to feel seen, catered for and healed, knowing that you are never alone in your experiences and the possibilities of contentment and progress are never far away.

This book might be the start of your healing journey or it may be a signal that you are on your way to being healed, although in truth it's no linear journey with a final destination. Either way, you are the one to decide, and that's a pretty poignant moment for us to let sink in.

Again, this is a guide and a book to be carried with us through the ages and hopefully from generation to generation, which, in itself, I hope will free us from the feeling of doom. Do not underestimate how far we have come. Yes, we have even further to go but it will hopefully be an easier ride than the ones who came before us, who bore us with the sole intention of moving our culture and our communities forward. We are living dreams and we are also living someone's dream. We must remember that and never forget it, even during tough times. We are living inspirations and we need to conserve that for ourselves at times too.

This book is a commitment to you, my legacy and a commitment to self. Treat it as such and let it comfort you in the similar ways it brought me peace. Now we are together, let's stay together and let's stay connected. Let me know what worked for you, if you've seen transformations after stepping into this book and my world, let me know your experiences – sharing this will bring us all closer and further forward as an intersection. DM me, comment on a post, write me an email, suggest a tea catch-up, regardless of what you decide is your best form of communicating that this book served you, I really want to know. And if you want more, scream it from the rooftops: the louder we are, the further we get – don't let anyone tell you otherwise. Loud, proud, Black. That's us.

And remember you are enough. Black women are enough. What we want is enough and those who persist will receive.

That's us.

ACKNOWLEDGEMENTS

Getting to this part of the writing feels like an accomplishment. I feel so full! To see this project to the end (or the end for now), to have collaborated with so many incredibly talented people and to be able to see my wildest dreams come to fruition is nothing short of phenomenal – although it is humbling, too. I have so many people to thank, but I want to start this with a line for the Almighty, my God. Without you, this opportunity and this book may have never materialised. You kept me going in my darkest of hours, when my world flipped upside down several times over and I honestly never thought I would be here and finalising one of the biggest projects of my life. Without you nothing is possible. Thank you for giving me my strength, my ideas, my skillset, for helping me find my power and reigniting my faith, my ability to create community and the ambition to keep going. Also thank you for my son, who I hope one day will be as proud of me for this project as you are.

Thank you to the people who made this book a reality. From the jump, Ebyan Egal, thank you for thinking of me and getting this concept over the line. Meeting you has been one of the greatest moments of my career. In a time of darkness for Black people across the world and especially women like you and I, you found strength, you found thy.self and you found me. To Katie Packer, my editor, you deserve all the flowers. Juggling your own blossoming career alongside me and my way of working, you are nothing short of the MVP I never knew I needed. Thank you for this opportunity, your time and sticking beside me. Thank you to Feyi and the Headline team for your tireless work.

To all who said yes without hesitation when asked to contribute to the book, you don't know how much I rate each and every one of you. Individually your tireless work towards the things and people that matter the most to you, inspire me to get up and do better every day. Without you, my career and life both on- and offline wouldn't even be nearly as close to exciting as it has been. Not many can say they know such a plethora of professional, classy, on-their-shit Black women as I can, who will willingly share their schedules to make this book happen, so this final product of love and effort is for you as much as it is for the community and the readers. Thank you, Enam Asiama, Char Ellesse, Paula Akpan, Agnes Mwakatuma, Aisha Carrington, Laurise McMillian, Natasha Sackey, the BAATN, Charlotte Williams, Natty Kasambala, Nicole Crentsil, Sharmaine Lovegrove, Diahann Holder and Aja Barber.

To Jocelyn, who isn't in this book but feels like she's with me all the time, thank you for your calm words, allowing me to be vulnerable yet safe and showing up in the pivotal moments of my life on Earth like the angel you are.

And to my incredibly supportive friends, who have lifted

Acknowledgements

me up and supported this project and me without question, through the many dark hours, I am so grateful for you and our friendship. Thank you to my non-Black female friends for recognising the importance of a book like this and for being the example the world needs for friendship and allyship. Stacy-Jayne Archer, Clancy Ferris and Claire James – I love you.

Huge thanks to all my internet friends and supporters who continue to like and share my work, especially with thy.self, in your personal and professional conversations. I respect and honour you more than you know. For those who have rooted for me and this project, I am very grateful and can feel the loving energy even when I can't pinpoint where exactly it's coming from. To anyone reading this, thank you!

And lastly, to the Black woman reading this and to the Black women that came before me, my icons, my 'competitors', my ancestors and 'the village', none of this would be possible without you. I said it in the beginning, and I will say it again, I couldn't have done this for anyone else. I exist, I am inspired, I will forever be a proud Black woman. I am proudly one of you. This is for us! May we be and see the change we are collectively working so hard for.